The book of Charmaine Husum is a valuable contribution to the important subject of integration and healing by building a bridge between the work with psychedelics and art therapy. As an art therapist with extensive experience with trauma work she is providing the theoretical background of psychedelic work and art therapy combined with practical creative exercises and meditations supporting the integration of experiences in non-ordinary states of consciousness. The use of art as an instrument of integration has been part of my psychedelic research since the early years in Prague, Czech Republic and is still an important part of my contemporary holotropic work and our training with breathwork (Grof ® Breathwork) and psychedelics www.grof-legacy-training.com. Her book on psychedelics and art therapy can offer important guidelines for the work of therapists and for anybody who wishes to use art therapy as an instrument to deepen the integration of psychedelic experiences.

Stanislav Grof, *MD, PHD, Author of* The Way of the Psychonaut
Brigitte Grof, *PhD, Author of* Holotropic Art-Images from Hidden Worlds

"*Psychedelics and Art Therapy* brings together two healing traditions in a clear, comprehensive and constructive way. It finds a nice balance between theoretical context and clinical practicality. It offers a unique blend of Art Therapy, meditation, and neuroscience, specifically tailored to the integration of Psychedelic experiences into daily life. As a workbook, it has an important place as an adjunct in working with a therapist and will be useful as a self-help guide for those seeking healing and growth on their own. But there's also food aplenty here for both beginning therapists and experienced veterans."

Bruce Tobin, *PhD, RCC, ATR(BC) founder of TheraPsil (2019)*
Advocacy for patient access to medical psilocybin, Charter &
Honorary Life Member BC Art Therapy Assn

"This groundbreaking book is a must read for therapists navigating the new frontiers of Art Therapy and Psychedelics. Husum has written a very readable comprehensive workbook on non-ordinary states of consciousness, Psychedelics, and the use of meditation, breath work, and specifically the value and role for Art Therapy in this field. Husum advocates for a safe trauma-informed approach, and she is exceedingly thoughtful

regarding the legal and ethical aspects within the larger historical and medical context of using drugs for healing, personal growth, and therapy. Husum is aware of the value and historical use of plants in sacred and healing practices and the impact of the current Psychedelic tourism has on Indigenous cultures. Charmaine Husum's book will be of value for therapists and practitioners who wish to integrate meditation and creative explorations in the field of Psychedelics."

Monica Carpendale, *BFA, DVATI, RCAT, BCATR, HLM,*
Professor Emeritus, Kutenai Art Therapy Institute

Psychedelics and Art Therapy

This book serves as a vital resource for clinicians, therapists, and individuals aiming to integrate their psychedelic experiences through the transformative practice of Art Therapy. Rooted in a Trauma-informed approach, *Psychedelics and Art Therapy: A Trauma-Informed Manual for Somatic Self Discovery* offers guidance on navigating the profound psychological and emotional shifts that often accompany such journeys.

This book combines creative exercises with meditation and neuroscientific insights to show how Art Therapy can effectively reroute neural pathways, fostering sustained emotional well-being and personal growth. In an era where the underground market of psychedelic therapy is often unsafe and commercially driven, this book advocates for a sustainable approach to healing that prevents habitual reliance on these substances. Authored by an Art Therapist with over a decade of specialized experience in psychedelic preparation and integration, this book transcends the underground stigmas associated with drug culture, offering a trusted path to healing grounded in therapeutic practices that honor transpersonal and Indigenous wisdom.

As the conversation around Psychedelics in therapy evolves, this essential guide provides a structured and compassionate approach to integration and healing, ensuring long-term personal empowerment and inner well-being.

Charmaine Husum is an Art Therapist, Somatic Counselor, and Kundalini yoga and meditation instructor specializing in supporting those healing from trauma and training others in using Art Therapy within the psychedelic healing space.

Psychedelics and Art Therapy

A Trauma-Informed Manual for Somatic Self-Discovery

Charmaine Husum

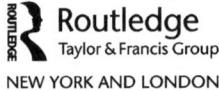
Routledge
Taylor & Francis Group

NEW YORK AND LONDON

Designed cover image: © Cover art created by Charmaine Husum
photographed by Michael Brager

First published 2025
by Routledge
605 Third Avenue, New York, NY 10158

and by Routledge
4 Park Square, Milton Park, Abingdon, Oxon, OX14 4RN

Routledge is an imprint of the Taylor and Francis Group, an informa business

© 2025 Charmaine Husum

Library of Congress Cataloging-in-Publication Data
Names: Husum, Charmaine, author.
Title: Psychedelics and art therapy: a trauma-informed manual for somatic
self-discovery / Charmaine Husum.
Description: New York, NY: Routledge, 2025. |
Includes bibliographical references and index.
Identifiers: LCCN 2024057989 (print) | LCCN 2024057990 (ebook) |
ISBN 9781032978468 (hardback) | ISBN 9781032975931 (paperback) |
ISBN 9781003595762 (ebook)
Subjects: MESH: Art Therapy | Hallucinogens—therapeutic use |
Psychological Trauma—drug therapy | Lysergic Acid Diethylamide—
therapeutic use
Classification: LCC RC489.A7 (print) | LCC RC489.A7 (ebook) |
NLM WM 450.5.A8 | DDC 616.89/1656—dc23/eng/20250317
LC record available at https://lccn.loc.gov/2024057989
LC ebook record available at https://lccn.loc.gov/2024057990

ISBN: 978-1-032-97846-8 (hbk)
ISBN: 978-1-032-97593-1 (pbk)
ISBN: 978-1-003-59576-2 (ebk)

DOI: 10.4324/9781003595762

Typeset in Adobe Caslon Pro by codeMantra

For Product Safety Concerns and Information please contact our EU representative:
GPSR@taylorandfrancis.com.
Taylor & Francis Verlag GmbH, Kaufingerstraße 24, 80331 München, Germany.

CONTENTS

PREFACE

The creation of this book is deeply intertwined with my own journey—a journey of transformation, healing, and the profound realization of how art, Psychedelics, and meditation, when applied together, can foster true lasting change. Through my experiences with Psychedelics, breathwork, and other non-ordinary states of consciousness (NOSC) to heal past trauma, I quickly realized that something was missing afterward. Often the ceremonies I attended would conclude with a brief circle where participants could share their experiences, but more often than not, there was little to no follow-up. While the importance of integration was becoming more recognized, the support offered was minimal, perhaps a phone call or virtual session weeks later. I found myself needing something more tangible—a felt internal experience expressed externally—something that would serve as a record of the wisdom I had received to fully process and integrate these experiences into my life.

By using Art Therapy in conjunction with somatic processes, or body awareness, we can create a shift in our lives that, for many, traditional talk therapy does not achieve. Short integration sessions after a NOSC experience weren't enough for me. As a result of not feeling fully integrated, I continued to look outside of myself for healing, which meant using the medicine again and again without fully integrating the profound wisdom I was given. Looking outside of oneself for healing is a pattern I've noticed with those who have used Psychedelic medicines for healing. I continually hear the phrase "Trust the Medicine" and although surrendering to the experience is part of the process, I believe lasting healing comes from developing a relationship with ourselves so that we can move forward in life, trusting our own inner wisdom, reignited by the medicine.

Art has always been a way to document, process, and make sense of non-ordinary states. In the context of psychedelic healing, art becomes a bridge between altered states of consciousness and the return to everyday life. It provides a structured yet deeply personal way to prepare for and integrate these experiences, turning fleeting insights into lasting change. Through art, the abstract, ineffable, and sometimes overwhelming experiences of Psychedelics can be grounded, understood, and ultimately transformed into a source of personal empowerment.

Often individuals reach for these medicines as a last resort—a hope for a magic bullet to overcome issues such as trauma, ongoing depression, Post-Traumatic Stress Disorder, anxiety, and other mental health issues. The importance of a Trauma-informed lens becomes imperative, yet given the intensity of these experiences, re-traumatization can occur, making proper preparation, integration, and connection to internal resources even more important.

What has fueled my passion further in working in this realm, supporting others on their healing journeys, are the tragic losses of friends and colleagues to suicide after using Psychedelics. These events highlighted the critical need for structured, supportive frameworks in preparing for and integrating psychedelic experiences. This book was born out of that need, combining my personal experiences, professional expertise, and a deep understanding of how art can facilitate healing.

This book, *Psychedelics and Art Therapy: A Trauma-Informed Guide to Somatic Self Discovery*, offers specific tools designed to help navigate this journey. My hope is that they will serve and support you, the reader, in learning new ways to prepare for and integrate NOSC. The power of art to transcend darkness, to connect us with ourselves and others, to reflect and reorient, and to heal has always been a part of the human experience. This book aims to show you how this modality of healing supports the further exploration and transformation that NOSC can bring.

In sharing the lessons I have learned, I hope to illuminate a path for others. This book is a guide for those searching for healing in their own lives. It is a testament to the power of art, the importance of proper preparation and integration of psychedelic experiences, and the deep connection between the sacred and the personal journey toward healing.

ACKNOWLEDGMENTS

With deep humility and gratitude, I honor the Indigenous peoples worldwide who have safeguarded and shared the wisdom of sacred medicines for generations. Their ancestral knowledge, rooted in reverence, reciprocity, and deep ecological wisdom, has profoundly shaped our understanding of healing, creativity, and transformation. I recognize the healers, knowledge keepers, and ancestors who have carried these traditions despite colonization, displacement, and erasure. Their resilience and generosity have paved the way for many to integrate these sacred practices into therapeutic and artistic work.

This book stands on the foundation of their wisdom. May we approach this work with respect, integrity, and a commitment to reciprocity—supporting Indigenous sovereignty, land stewardship, and the rights of traditional medicine carriers. I also acknowledge the lands on which this book was written and their original caretakers. May we continue to listen, learn, and honor these teachings with the care they deserve.

To all those who believed in me when I struggled to believe in myself—thank you. Mr. Gary Robertson, my high school art teacher, your encouragement gave me the courage to find my voice through art. Millie Cumming, my professor in graduate school, your wisdom and kindness guided me through the complexities of becoming an Art Therapist and shaped the foundation of my professional path. I am deeply grateful to the many mentors and teachers who have given their time, energy, and resources to support my growth. Your guidance has been invaluable, and your belief in me has propelled me forward in ways words cannot fully express.

To the unseen forces that have walked with me—my guardian angels, my grandmother, my ancestors, and the spirit of the medicines—you have guided and protected me through every step of this journey. Your presence is felt in the deepest moments of healing, and I honor you with gratitude.

Finally, to those who have suffered in silence and to those who have lost their lives after not having the proper support following psychedelic experiences—this book is for you. Your stories are woven into the fabric of this work, and your courage has inspired me to create something that I hope will help others find the support they need. Thank you.

DISCLAIMER AND INFORMED CONSENT

Disclaimer

This program uses a harm-reduction integration approach to psychedelic healing and in no way promotes, condones, or facilitates illegal activity. Although we are in a Psychedelic Renaissance with clinical trials being conducted around the world, please be aware that psychedelic substances still remain illegal in many countries.

This book is intended to support you, or those you support, on a journey toward integration and is not intended to replace medical intervention.

By reading the content in this book, you are agreeing that Charmaine Husum at the Centre of the Heart takes no responsibilities for your actions.

Informed Consent

This book is designed to provide education from our personal and professional experiences. Please be aware that it is for educational purposes only. This is not a substitute for traditional psychotherapy or medicine. If you are experiencing significant issues, please seek medical attention.

Limitations of the Material in This Book

The exercises in this book are oriented toward personal and spiritual development. The techniques or modalities are in no way a replacement for traditional therapy but meant to support you, or those you support. If you are needing additional support, please reach out for individual private counseling sessions.

INTRODUCTION

Have you found yourself grappling to make sense of a profound experience? Perhaps you feel that only the surface has been touched, and you're yearning to delve deeper into understanding yourself and how to truly live your best life.

The effects of altered states of consciousness ripple through our waking reality far beyond the initial ceremony or circumstances that brought us there. Whether your journey has been through sacred plant medicines or entheogens like Ayahuasca, Psilocybin, or Iboga; synthetic Psychedelics such as LSD, MDMA, and Ketamine; or other consciousness-expanding experiences like a Kundalini Awakening, Dark Night of the Soul, Meditation, or Yoga, a profound shift occurs in both the body and brain. Returning to regular waking life can often feel confusing after such transformative experiences.

My name is Charmaine Husum, and I specialize in helping people understand and integrate their psychedelic experiences using Trauma-informed Art Therapy, counseling, meditation, and connecting with the innate wisdom of the body. My personal journey with breathwork and Psychedelics for deeper self-awareness left me with more questions than answers. Initially, I thought I needed more medicine, more ceremonies—more insights from outside myself—to further decipher my experiences. This was counterintuitive to my knowledge as a therapist—that lasting healing comes from within. This realization made the importance of integration crystal clear; the answers I needed were already awakened by those earlier psychedelic experiences and were waiting within me!

This book is intended to deepen your relationship with the healing you are about to, or have already, touched upon with Psychedelics. It invites you to explore and integrate your Soul-awakening experience by nurturing the inherent wisdom that has always lived within you. Throughout these pages, an opened portal awaits, inviting expanded learning as the natural wisdom of your body and mind integrate your experiences into lasting life changes on your healing journey.

My approach to integration is through a Trauma-informed lens, an essential perspective, as past traumas often surface for healing during non-ordinary states. The protocols I have developed support a deepened process within the stages of psychedelic therapy or a non-ordinary state of consciousness (NOSC). This book follows the three-stage trauma healing model first outlined by Judith Herman (1992); a framework widely used by trauma therapists. You will also explore new ways of being in the world by incorporating recent discoveries from neuroscience and neuroplasticity, examining your dreams, your artwork, calming the nervous system through meditation and yoga, and tapping into the innate wisdom of the body to learn tools that will help you thrive in life.

By understanding the neuroscientific restructuring that occurs in the brain during non-ordinary states, we will harness the benefits of Art Therapy and meditation, which similarly create and strengthen new neural pathways to support integration. Exploring your spiritual relationship with the experience and deepening this connection through reflection and meditation will lead to lasting changes that will continue to shape your life for years to come.

The goal is to make sense of what happened so that you are in control of the shift this experience has presented to you—allowing you to create the life you have always intended. Enjoy the journey; it will be memorable.

ABOUT THE AUTHOR

Charmaine Husum RCAT, RTC, CT, DKATI is a registered Art Therapist, somatic counsellor, Kundalini yoga teacher, and psychedelic integration specialist, whose work is deeply rooted in the intersection of creativity, healing, and spiritual connection. With nearly 30 years of professional artistic experience, Charmaine's journey began as an internationally recognized scenic artist, contributing to major film and television productions such as *Brokeback Mountain, Twilight, The Imaginarium of Dr. Parnassus, Night at the Museum,* and *The Last of Us.* Her artistic talents led her to work with some of the most prominent creative geniuses of our time, including Tom Waits and directors such as Terry Gilliam and Ang Lee, crafting immersive environments that have been celebrated on both screen and stage.

However, it is her personal journey through trauma and healing that has most profoundly shaped her career. From an early age, she found solace and expression in art, dance, and poetry—tools that helped her navigate the challenges of abuse, foster care, leaving home at 14, and overcoming early escapism through self-harm, drugs, and alcohol. These personal experiences with the transformative power of creative expression laid the foundation for her later work as an Art Therapist.

After extensive travel and living in different parts of the world, Charmaine now runs her private practice, *Centre of the HeArt,* on the traditional territories of the Blackfoot Confederacy (Siksika, Kainai, and Piikani), the Tsuut'ina, the Îyâxe Nakoda Nations, and the Métis people of Calgary, Alberta, Canada. Here, she offers both in-person and online support to clients regionally and internationally, helping them integrate the insights and healing gained from their lived and psychedelic experiences through Trauma-informed Art Therapy, counseling, meditation, and somatic approaches.

Her current research delves into the exciting fields of neuroplasticity, neuroscience, epigenetics, and mystical/psychedelic integration, exploring how ancestral experiences influence our lives today. Charmaine's belief that the traumas and stories of our ancestors are encoded in our DNA fuels her passion for helping others heal not just themselves but also the generational wounds that may linger within.

Although her extensive experimentation with Psychedelics began recreationally at a very young age, the transformational healing she experienced was only achieved through structured ceremony, later on in life. Her own work using psychedelic plant medicines and breathwork for healing, revealed to her a distressing gap within the potential of lasting transformation when proper integration and follow-up support wasn't available. Ceremonies could leave her feeling empty and without the answers needed as she looked outside of herself for healing. Her training in Art Therapy and deep meditation allowed for true healing and to make sense of the wisdom received during ceremonies.

As she continued working within the subculture of psychedelic therapy, the shadow sides that could emerge without proper preparation and integration became increasingly apparent. After experiencing and hearing numerous accounts of people ending their lives after using medicines intended for healing, her commitment to supporting the preparation and integration of Psychedelics became a mission—one fueled by her own transformative experiences with Art Therapy and Meditation. This fire continues to burn brightly, refusing to be extinguished.

Contrary to many working in this field, Charmaine does not advocate for the use of Psychedelics but rather the support of proper preparation and integration and believes that true and lasting healing can only come from within.

As an advocate for a harm-reduction and Trauma-informed approach in the therapeutic use of Psychedelics, for more than a decade, Charmaine has labored over the creation of this book *Psychedelics and Art Therapy: A Trauma-Informed Manual for Somatic Self Discovery* and created the Psychedelics and Art Therapy— Preparation and Integration course, aimed at providing structured, supportive frameworks for individuals to process and integrate their psychedelic journeys. She is committed to helping her clients tap into their inner resources and transpersonal connections to spirit after experiencing non-ordinary states of consciousness, whether through Psychedelics or other means.

Through her workshops, trainings and international retreats, Charmaine continues to share her knowledge and expertise, guiding others on their paths to healing and personal growth. Her visionary art, which she describes as channeling energy beyond herself, stands as a testament to her belief that beauty can emerge from hardship and that creative expression is a profound catalyst for transformation.

For more information about Charmaine's work or to book an individual session, visit www.centreoftheheart.com.

PART I
LAYING THE FOUNDATION

As many of you may be aware, we are currently experiencing a renaissance in the use of Psychedelics in healing and mental health. Research is abundant with findings on the benefits and impacts these substances have on the brain and long-term psychological well-being. Yet, despite professionals in the field continuing to emphasize the importance of integration and cautioning against repercussions when integration is not therapeutically supported, one crucial aspect of this process has largely been left out of mainstream discussions: Art and the indispensable role Art Therapy needs to play in Psychedelic Therapy.

From the ancient wisdom of Indigenous peoples to thought leaders in psychology, processing altered states through artistic expression has always been a part of the conversation. In this book, we delve into the profound connection between art, transpersonal experiences, and the use of psychedelic medicines while exploring the role Art Therapy can play in this dynamic exchange. A focus on recent research into the neuroscience of Psychedelics will be explored as we learn tools for rerouting neural pathways within the brain through Therapeutic Art Interventions, Meditation, Journaling, and the Exploration of Dreams.

Through a Trauma-informed and harm-reduction lens, the teachings in this book facilitate a more complete integration of psychedelic

DOI: 10.4324/9781003595762-1

experiences, ensuring that the wisdom gained in ceremony becomes an integral part of everyday life. By combining the tools of Art Therapy with Psychedelic-Assisted Therapy (PAT), we address challenges that may arise from inadequate preparation and integration, such as when the journey triggers trauma, when "bad trips" or challenging content emerge, when insights from the journey are not translated into actionable sources and strategies for change, and most importantly, when one develops a dependency on heightened states of consciousness to experience a sense of well-being.

This book is designed for individuals who have experienced Psychedelics, guides, and mental health professionals. It demonstrates that possessing the right tools, particularly through artistic interventions and mindfulness, are essential for comprehensive therapeutic support in the use of Psychedelics. In the midst of the ongoing psychedelic renaissance, overlooking the pivotal role of art and Art Therapy in this new era would be a significant oversight. As this revolution continues to unfold, incorporating ethical and effective art interventions into the discussion becomes imperative for the advancement of Psychedelic Assisted Therapy.

1
WHAT IS ART THERAPY?

Art Therapy is a mental health profession that leverages the creative process to enhance the physical, mental, and emotional well-being of individuals across all age groups. This therapeutic approach integrates psychotherapeutic techniques with art-making to improve mental health and overall well-being. Sometimes referred to as "Creative Arts Therapy" or "Expressive Arts Therapy," Art Therapy is grounded in the belief that the creative process involved in artistic self-expression helps people resolve conflicts and problems, develop interpersonal skills, manage behavior, reduce stress, increase self-esteem and self-awareness, and achieve insight.

The profession of Art Therapy integrates the fields of human development, visual arts (including drawing, painting, sculpture, and other art forms), and the creative process with models of counseling and psychotherapy. Art Therapy is used to assess and treat a wide range of conditions, including but not limited to:

- Anxiety, depression, and other mental and emotional problems and disorders
- Impulsivity and attentional issues like ADHD and Autism
- Substance abuse and other addictions
- Family and relationship issues

DOI: 10.4324/9781003595762-2

- Abuse and domestic violence
- Social and emotional difficulties related to disability and illness
- Trauma and loss
- Physical, cognitive, and neurological problems
- Psychosocial difficulties

Art Therapy also supports those seeking to enhance their quality of life, support relaxation and self-care, move creative blocks, and explore aspects of creativity.

Key Figures in Art Therapy: Origins and Future Directions

The concept of using art in psychotherapy has deep historical roots, but it gained significant prominence in the early 20th century with psychoanalysts like Carl Jung, who integrated artistic expression into therapeutic practice. Jung was one of the first to utilize art as a tool for exploring the unconscious mind. His work with mandalas, for instance, provided a pathway for individuals to delve into their inner worlds, facilitating a sense of psychological wholeness. Jung's approach laid an early foundation for the use of art within a therapeutic context, inspiring future practitioners.

Margaret Naumburg, often hailed as the "mother of Art Therapy," was pivotal in formalizing the field in the early 20th century. Building on Jung's concepts, Naumburg introduced the idea of artistic expression as a means of accessing unconscious thoughts and emotions, much like the way dreams operate. She integrated art as a central component of her therapeutic practice, establishing a distinct approach that would become the bedrock of modern Art Therapy. Her innovative work emphasized the power of spontaneous creation, allowing clients to express emotions and gain insights without the constraints of verbal language.

Florence Cane, Naumburg's sister and colleague, expanded upon this notion by focusing on the creative process itself as a therapeutic tool. Cane's techniques encouraged spontaneous and intuitive art-making, which she believed could reveal inner conflicts and facilitate emotional release. By prioritizing the act of creation over interpretative analysis, she opened the door for individuals to explore their psyche in a direct, non-verbal way.

Edith Kramer further developed the field by highlighting the healing potential inherent in the creative process. Unlike previous approaches that focused on interpreting the final artwork, Kramer emphasized that the very act of making art could foster personal insight and emotional healing. Her contributions underscored the importance of the creative process in therapy, reinforcing the idea that artistic expression could serve as a vehicle for self-discovery and psychological integration.

Art Therapy has continued to grow and evolve, drawing on recent discoveries in neuroscience and neuroplasticity. This ongoing evolution aligns with the foundational work of early pioneers, who recognized the value of art as a means of accessing emotions that are difficult to articulate. Today, Art Therapy offers a non-verbal outlet for expression, enabling individuals to access and express parts of themselves that may lie beyond the reach of words. As the field advances, the contributions of these key figures continue to inform and shape its practices, pointing towards an increasingly integrative and holistic future for Art Therapy.

Ethical Considerations in Art Therapy and the Importance of Professional Training

In the growing field of psychedelic-assisted therapy, Art Therapy has emerged as a powerful tool for self-expression, exploration, and integration of psychedelic experiences. However, while engaging with art as a means of therapy can be deeply transformative, it also carries significant ethical considerations. In this section, we will explore the importance of ethical practice in Art Therapy, especially in the context of Psychedelics, and discuss why it is crucial for a trained and certified Art Therapist to facilitate these processes. It is essential to clarify upfront that this book is neither a substitute for professional training nor a manual to train individuals as Art Therapists. Instead, it aims to offer supportive directives for personal exploration while acknowledging the necessity of consulting a qualified Art Therapist when needed.

The Ethical Landscape of Art Therapy

Art Therapy sits at the intersection of psychological exploration and creative expression. This dual nature requires careful ethical considerations. The process of creating art can evoke powerful emotions, memories, and insights, especially when combined with the altered states of consciousness induced by Psychedelics. In this vulnerable space, ethical practices ensure the safety and well-being of the individual.

Art Therapy involves a set of guiding principles such as confidentiality, informed consent, professional boundaries, and respect for the client's autonomy. These principles are designed to protect individuals as they navigate potentially intense emotional experiences. In psychedelic-assisted therapy, where the boundaries of consciousness are expanded, it becomes even more vital to adhere to these ethical standards.

When untrained individuals attempt to facilitate Art Therapy without understanding these ethical nuances, they risk causing harm. For example, a lack of awareness about Trauma-informed practices can lead to the unintentional re-traumatization of individuals who may encounter distressing memories or feelings during their art-making process. Thus, ensuring that Art Therapy is conducted ethically and with proper training is not only a professional obligation but also a moral imperative.

The Importance of Professional Training in Art Therapy

A trained Art Therapist is equipped with the knowledge and skills necessary to guide individuals through complex psychological landscapes safely. Art Therapists are trained to create a supportive environment, assess the client's needs, and adapt interventions to suit the individual's emotional state and therapeutic goals. This level of expertise is especially crucial in the context of Psychedelics, where experiences can be unpredictable and profoundly impactful.

Professional training in Art Therapy involves extensive education in both the therapeutic and artistic aspects of the practice. Art Therapists learn how to facilitate various art-making processes, interpret the symbolic content of art, and navigate the therapeutic relationship ethically. They are trained to understand the psychological and neurological processes involved in both art-making and altered states of consciousness. This knowledge allows them to support clients in integrating their experiences into a coherent narrative that promotes healing and growth.

Moreover, trained Art Therapists are skilled in identifying when additional clinical interventions are necessary. For instance, if a client begins to exhibit signs of severe distress or trauma during their art-making process, a professional can recognize these signals and provide the appropriate support. In cases where the individual's needs surpass the scope of Art Therapy, the therapist can refer them to other mental health professionals or complementary therapeutic modalities.

Consulting an Art Therapist: When Is It Needed?

While this book offers suggestions and directives that can support your personal exploration of art and Psychedelics, it is important to emphasize that these are not a replacement for professional Art Therapy. Engaging in art-making as part of self-care or self-reflection can be beneficial; however, it does not equate to the depth and safety provided by a structured therapeutic process led by a trained professional.

Consulting an Art Therapist may be especially necessary in the following scenarios:

1. **Processing Trauma:** If your psychedelic experiences bring up traumatic memories or feelings that you find difficult to process alone, it is crucial to seek the support of a trained Art Therapist. They can help you navigate these emotions in a way that fosters healing rather than re-traumatization.

2. **Severe Emotional Distress:** Should you experience intense emotional reactions during your self-guided Art Therapy, such as overwhelming anxiety, depression, or existential fear, a professional Art Therapist can provide the necessary tools and techniques to help you manage these feelings.

3. **Integration of Complex Psychedelic Experiences:** Psychedelic experiences can sometimes be profound, multilayered, and challenging to interpret. An Art Therapist can assist in unpacking these experiences, facilitating integration in a manner that supports long-term personal growth.

4. **Desire for Structured Therapeutic Support:** If you wish to engage in art-making within a structured, therapeutic framework that addresses specific psychological or emotional issues, consulting a trained Art Therapist ensures you receive guidance tailored to your unique needs.

Supporting Your Personal Process: The Scope of This Book

The directives and exercises offered in this book are meant to support you in your own exploration of art-making as part of your psychedelic journey. They are designed to encourage self-reflection, creativity, personal expression while supporting and promoting healing and growth. However, it is essential to reiterate that these suggestions do not replace clinical interventions or the role of a trained Art Therapist.

Art Therapy is a nuanced practice that requires both knowledge and sensitivity to the client's psychological state. The safety and effectiveness of Art Therapy in the context of Psychedelics rely on the therapist's ability to hold space, provide guidance, and ensure ethical practice throughout the process. While this book aims to empower you in your personal journey, it is important to seek professional support when the complexities of your experiences call for it.

In the journey of self-discovery through art and Psychedelics, recognize when it is time to seek the guidance of a professional. Doing so not only honors your own process but also respects the transformative power of Art Therapy, ensuring it serves as a positive force in your healing and integration.

2
THEORY AND HISTORY OF ART AND NON-ORDINARY STATES

What Is a Non-Ordinary State?

A non-ordinary state of consciousness (NOSC) refers to an altered state of awareness that differs from our everyday waking consciousness. These states can be induced through various means, such as meditation, breathwork, ritual, dance, prayer, near death experiences or the use of psychoactive substances. In non-ordinary states, individuals may experience shifts in perception, cognition, and sense of self.

Ancient Practices

Throughout history, artists, mystics, and shamans have explored non-ordinary states through various means. Art has been and is still used as a tool for expressing, documenting, and exploring the mysteries of the human psyche and the cosmos. It connects us to feeling states beyond conscious thought. Dating as far back as 36,000 years, cave art found in France, Siberia, Mesoamerica, South Africa, Algeria, and California, proves that ineffable experiences are best described and processed with an expression that utilizes the creative process. Art from ancient Egypt, Greece, medieval and renaissance paintings also exemplify that art has always been an important part of processing non-ordinary states of consciousness (NOSC). Some examples include

DOI: 10.4324/9781003595762-3

Lascaux Cave Paintings (France)

The famous Lascaux cave paintings in France's Dordogne region show-case various animals and abstract forms. Some scholars suggest that they might have been created during altered states of consciousness, indi-cating the spiritual practices of ancient humans. These artworks are an important part of prehistoric art, highlighting the deep bond between humans and nature.

Chauvet Cave Paintings (France)

The Chauvet Cave, discovered in 1994, contains some of the oldest known figurative cave paintings, dating back around 36,000 years. The famous Panel of Lions, located deep within the cave, is one of the most significant artworks. Some experts suggest that the artist may have been influenced by hypoxia—lack of oxygen—leading to hallucinations that inspired the creation of these intricate and haunting images. These art-works provide insight into the early human experience and their connec-tion to the natural world.

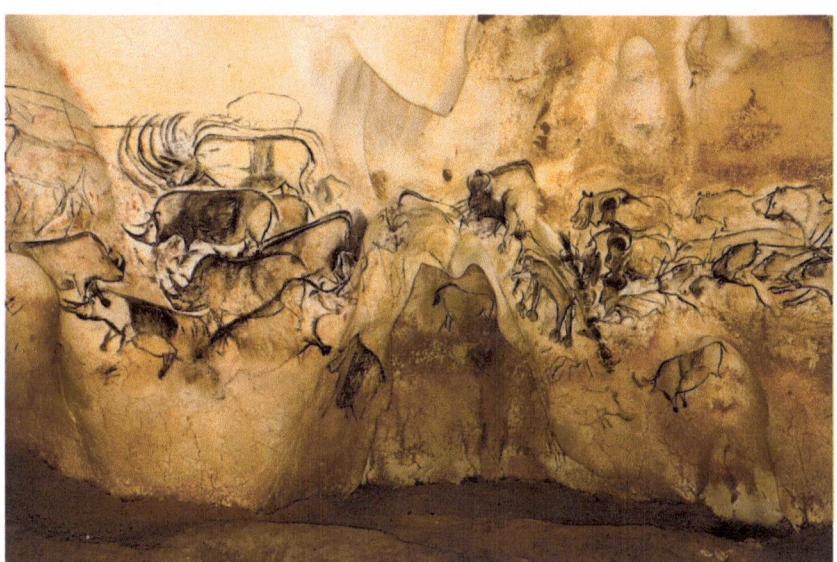

Figure 2.1 Chauvet Cave Paintings (France): Panel of Lions. Centre National De Préhistoire. Ministère De La Culture Et De La Communication. Photo by: J. Clottes Crédit: Ministère de la Culture: Rhinoceroses and Lions Panel, Back Room. Site: Grotte Chauvet-Pont-d'Arc (Ardèche), France

San Rock Art (Southern Africa)

The San rock art in the Drakensberg Mountains of South Africa is believed to depict trance dances and shamanistic rituals. The most important San ritual was the healing or trance dance where people would stomp and dance around a campfire for hours, clapping and singing songs of the tribe. These dances continue to be practiced amongst San groups living in the Kalahari today. Ancient paintings they created offer a window into the spiritual life of the San people, illustrating their rituals where dancers enter altered states of consciousness, connecting them to the spirit realm.

Indigenous American Rock Art

In North America, prehistoric Indigenous rock art is often linked to hallucinogenic experiences. Located near the edge of the traditional territory of the Chumash people, this cavern had been dubbed Pinwheel Cave after the swirling red painting on its curved ceiling. Recent research suggests that these artworks were part of communal rituals involving the use of hallucinogenic plants, reflecting the integral role of these practices in the daily and spiritual lives of these communities. Here we have a representation thought to represent the flowers of *Datura wrightii*, a plant historically used for its hallucinogenic properties as part of elaborate community ceremonies, highlighting the deep appreciation of hallucinogenic plants for native Californian people. Found in the late 1990s by staff of the Wind Wolves Preserve (the owner of the land), researchers also discovered a number of chewed materials, which were almost all found to be made from the plant Datura. Datura flowers found in Native California were historically known to be a part of adolescent initiations, where young people would drink the processed root of the plant.

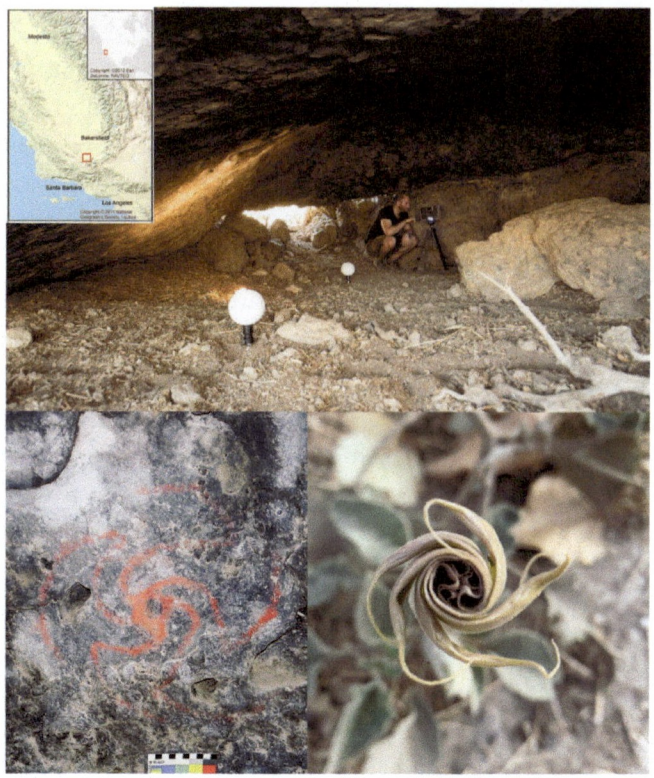

Figure 2.2 Indigenous American Rock Art. (Bottom Left) Pinwheel painting within the cave. Image credit: Rick Bury (photographer). (Bottom Right) Unfurling flower of *D. wrightii* from a plant near cave site. Image credit: Melissa Dabulamanzi (photographer). (Top Image) Expedition locating chewed plant matter near site of the hallucinogenic plant seen in lower photos. Permission by David Wayne Robinson, University of Central Lancashire

Tassili n'Ajjer Cave Art (Algeria)

The cave paintings at Tassili n'Ajjer, dating back to around 4,700 BC, illustrate shamans taking part in rituals that include the use of psychedelic mushrooms. These paintings are some of the earliest known representations of psychedelic use in spiritual practices in ancient North Africa. Ethnobotanist Terence McKenna describes these scenes in his book, *Food of the Gods: The Search for the Original Tree of Knowledge* (1993). He explains that the shamans are shown dancing, their hands filled with mushrooms, with others even appearing to grow from their bodies. In one depiction, the shamans are seen joyfully running, surrounded by intricate geometric patterns, likely representing their hallucinatory experiences. McKenna views this as strong visual evidence of early psychedelic use.

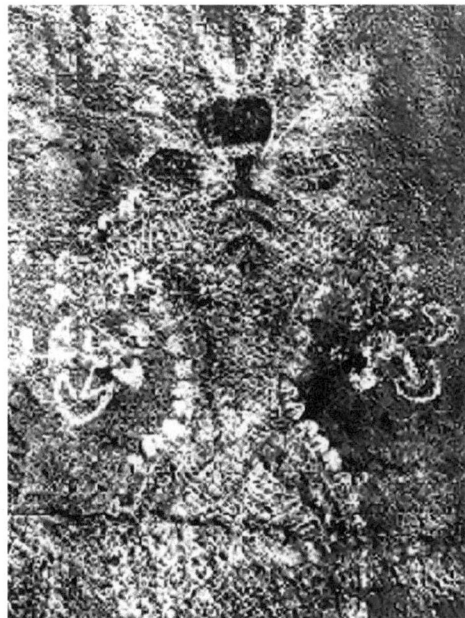

Figure 2.3 Tassili n'Ajjer Cave Art (Algeria). From the original photograph by Lajoux (1963)

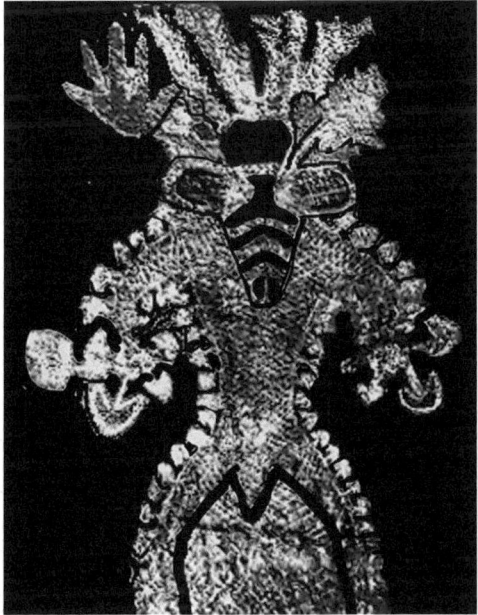

Figure 2.4 Tassili n'Ajjer Cave Art (Algeria). Outlined to clearly depict the image. From the original photograph by Lajoux (1963).

Eastern Spain Cave Art

Selva Pascuala is an ancient archaeological site located in eastern Spain, with carbon dating indicating its age to be between 6,000 and 8,000 years old. Archaeologists first uncovered this site in 1918, revealing a prehistoric mural painted on rock that depicts both mushrooms and a bull. It is one of about two dozen similar sites featuring Mesolithic to Neolithic rock art in the Mediterranean region of Spain. Upon comparing the local mushroom species with those depicted in the artwork, researchers have identified *Psilocybe hispanica* as a likely candidate, hinting at the possibility of psychoactive fungi being used in post-Paleolithic rituals.

Siberian Whale Hunter Cave Art

Archaeologists from the Institute of Archaeology RAS are urgently working to preserve ancient rock carvings depicting 'magic mushroom whale-hunting' people at Pegtymel, Chukotka, the northernmost art gallery in Eurasia. These images date back approximately 2,000 years. Located in an extremely remote region roughly 5,555 km east of Moscow, accessible only by helicopter, the cave art was created by nomadic whale hunters. Russian researchers have named the figures depicted as 'fly agaric people,' after the type of psychedelic mushrooms common in that area. Currently, efforts are being made to safeguard these unique rock images, now recognized as portrayals of ancient 'magic mushroom whale-hunters.'

The Art of Ancient Mesoamerican Cultures

The art of ancient Mesoamerican cultures, including the Maya and Aztec, often depicted shamanistic practices involving Psychedelics. Artifacts such as mushroom-human stone figurines and murals from Teotihuacan reveal the deep spiritual connection these cultures had with these substances.

Indigenous Australian Art

Dreamtime paintings, which represent the spiritual beliefs of Indigenous Australians, can be viewed in various galleries such as the National Gallery of Australia. These paintings depict creation myths and the spiritual connection of Indigenous Australians with their land. Dreams also represent an altered state, and using art to represent this state is another example of why art is so important when looking at ways to process, make sense of, and document NOSC.

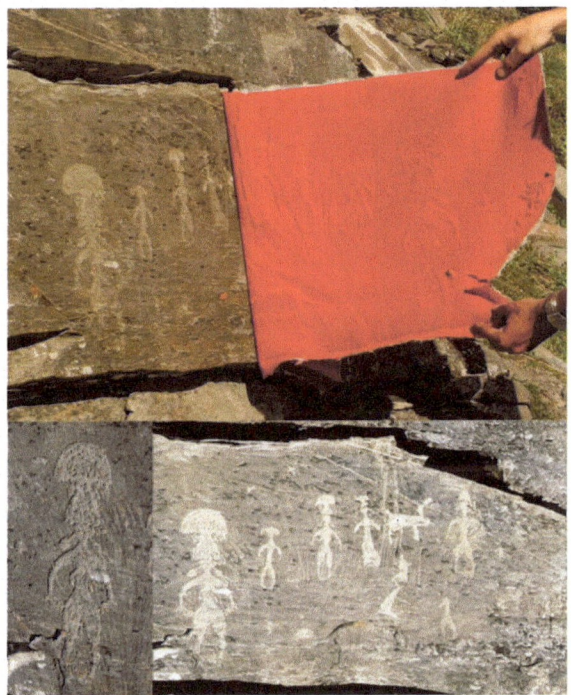

Figure 2.5 Siberian Whale Hunter Cave Art. Photo credit: Anthropomorphic figures in mushroom-shaped headdresses obtained with permission by https://archaeolog.ru/ru/about/history/expeditions-1990-present/20052008-gg--issledovaniya-naskalnykh-izobrazheniy-na-r-pegtymel-na-chukotke

Ancient Greek Art

The Eleusinian Mysteries, celebrated in reverence to the goddess Demeter and her daughter Persephone, held a sacred place in Ancient Greek religion, transcending the ordinary realm of worship. These mysteries were not merely rituals but profound experiences that blurred the lines between reality and the divine, drawing participants into a heightened state of consciousness.

Though much about the rites remain shrouded in mystery, it is believed that participants embarked on a symbolic journey along the Sacred Way, a pilgrimage that spanned ten days. This procession, marked by fasting and reflection, prepared the initiates for a transformative experience. Upon reaching the Temple of Demeter in Eleusis, they partook in Kykeon, a sacred drink whose very essence was believed to open the doors of perception.

This moment, when the participants consumed Kykeon, was not just an act of devotion but a gateway to an altered state of consciousness. In this heightened state, the boundaries of Self dissolved, and the initiates became one with the divine. They would then dance ecstatically, their movements embodying the myth of Demeter and Persephone, merging the sacred and the artistic in a vivid re-enactment.

Through this ritual, art became more than a medium—it was a living experience, a transformative act that allowed participants to connect deeply with the mythic and the transcendent, exploring the depths of human consciousness and its capacity for divine insight. Many artifacts were found from these ancient times, highlighting again how documenting these experiences gives them life and a story that can be understood and retold.

Renaissance and Baroque Art

Paintings by artists like Caravaggio depicting saints' ecstasies can be seen at the Galleria Borghese in Rome and in galleries around the world. Titled, Saint Francis of Assisi in Ecstasy," depicts the Cardinal's name-saint at the moment of receiving the signs of the Stigmata, the wounds left in Christ's body by the Crucifixion. This painting is just one example of an artist's depiction of an altered state. NOSC can be experienced through a multitude of means, prayer and deep meditation being just one of the many. These experiences have been portrayed in various art forms throughout the ages.

Islamic Art

Islamic art and architecture, known for their vibrant colors and intricate patterns, are often compared to the visuals experienced during psychedelic experiences. These artworks, such as those found in the Nasir al-Mulk Mosque in Shiraz, Iran, reflect the spiritual and mystical traditions of the Islamic world.

These examples illustrate that the rich history of NOSC across different cultures and periods would not be possible without creative processes. It validates and is a testament to why art is inherently linked to the use of psychedelic medicines and should continue.

3

TRANSPERSONAL PSYCHOLOGY, PSYCHEDELICS, AND ART

Transpersonal psychology and the study of creativity delve deeply into the fascinating relationship between art and non-ordinary states of consciousness. This field of psychology incorporates our connection to etheric concepts, like God, Source Energy, spiritual realms, the Soul, angels, etc. as a means of understanding and connecting deeper to the Self. Transpersonal psychology naturally lends itself to utilizing art as a way to explore and understand various realms of human consciousness more deeply. This is especially effective when combined with psychedelic experiences, which are often described as out-of-body experiences.

Stanislav Grof, one of the pioneering figures in transpersonal psychology, conducted extensive research into the effects of Psychedelics. He began his research with LSD (lysergic acid diethylamide), a powerful psychedelic drug that enhances thoughts, emotions, and sensory perception, in the mid-1950s at the Psychiatric Research Institute in Prague. His work extended into the 1960s, exploring the therapeutic potential of LSD and other psychedelic substances. In 1967, Grof moved to the United States, where he continued his research at Johns Hopkins University and later at the Maryland Psychiatric Research Center. Grof's work is foundational in understanding how altered states of consciousness can be therapeutic.

In addition to his work with LSD, Grof co-developed Holotropic Breathwork with his wife, Christina Grof, in the 1970s. Holotropic

DOI: 10.4324/9781003595762-4

Breathwork is a powerful technique that uses accelerated breathing, evocative music, and focused bodywork to access altered states of consciousness. This method allows individuals to explore the depths of their psyche and facilitate personal growth and healing without the use of Psychedelics.

Joan Kellogg, an Art Therapist, collaborated with Grof in examining the imagery and symbolism in art created by individuals under the influence of Psychedelics. Kellogg's contributions included the development of the "Mandala Assessment Research Instrument" (MARI), which used mandalas to understand and assess the psychological states of individuals. Her work highlighted the therapeutic potential of combining psychedelic experiences with artistic expression, allowing for deeper insight and integration of these experiences. Their studies revealed that psychedelic experiences often manifest in rich, symbolic art, reflecting profound psychological and spiritual insights.

Grof's work was significantly influenced by Carl Jung, a Swiss psychiatrist known for his theories of the collective unconscious. Jung posited that humans share universal archetypes and symbols, such as the mandala, which represents wholeness, unity, and completion. These symbols, deeply embedded in the human psyche, emerge vividly in art created during altered states, providing a window into universal human experiences and collective understanding.

In the 1950s and 1960s, Oscar Janiger, another key figure in the study of Psychedelics, was a pioneering psychiatrist and researcher in psychedelic therapy. Janiger is best known for his extensive research on the effects of LSD, particularly in relation to creativity. He famously conducted a study where he administered LSD to artists and then analyzed the impact on their creative output. His findings indicated that while Psychedelics enhanced creative thinking and expression, they could sometimes interfere with the technical execution of making art. Janiger's work was pivotal in highlighting the potential of Psychedelics to unlock creative potentials and alter perception in ways that foster artistic innovation.

Marlene Dobkin de Rios, an anthropologist and psychotherapist, made significant contributions to the understanding of Psychedelics and their cultural contexts. Conducting fieldwork in the Amazon for almost 30 years, starting in the late 1960s, she studied the use of entheogenic plants by the Indigenous peoples of Peru. Her research provided profound insights into how these communities use plant medicines like ayahuasca for healing, spiritual growth, and communal bonding. Dobkin de Rios's work emphasized the importance of cultural context in the use of Psychedelics and underscored the deep connection between entheogenic plant use and traditional healing practices. Her contributions helped bridge the gap between Western scientific approaches and Indigenous knowledge systems, enriching the broader understanding of Psychedelics.

Together, Oscar Janiger and Marlene Dobkin de Rios explored the intersections of art, Psychedelics, and cultural practices. They collaborated on studies that examined how the ingestion of LSD influenced the creative processes of artists. Their joint research included observing and analyzing the artwork produced by artists under the influence of Psychedelics. This collaboration helped to underscore the potential of Psychedelics to enhance creativity while also providing a deeper understanding of how different cultural contexts and personal histories can shape the psychedelic experience.

These researchers collectively highlight the profound relationship between art and Psychedelics. Their work underscores the importance of using art within psychedelic therapy as a means to access, explore, and integrate the powerful insights gained during altered states of consciousness. Art serves as a powerful tool to bridge the internal and external worlds, facilitating deeper self-understanding, healing, and transformation. By incorporating artistic expression into psychedelic therapy, individuals can harness the full potential of these experiences, promoting lasting psychological and spiritual growth.

4

PSYCHEDELIC ART

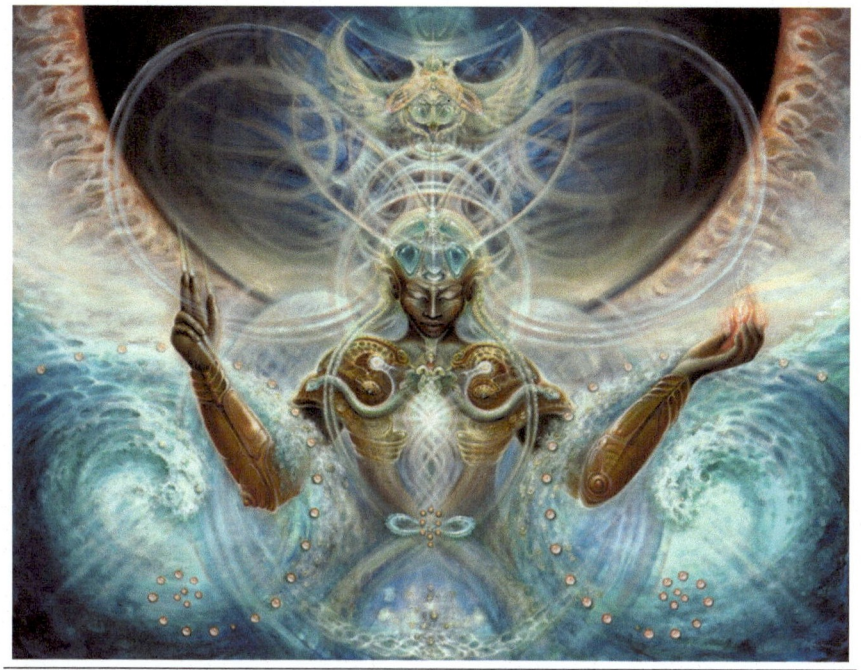

Figure 4.1 Image credit: THE BLESSING, Martina Hoffmann ©, 2024, Oil on Canvas

  DOI: 10.4324/9781003595762-5

Psychedelic art—art that is inspired by, influenced by, or derives from Psychedelics or non-ordinary states of consciousness—often captures the visual intensity, mystery, beauty, and sense of transcendence that can be experienced in altered states of consciousness. This unique form of art serves as a profound tool for integration, allowing individuals to process and express their psychedelic experiences in a tangible form. It is important to mention, that although therapeutic for the artist and viewer alike, psychedelic art differs from Art Therapy in specific elements.

Intent and Focus:

- **Psychedelic Art:** Focuses on aesthetic and expressive aspects, capturing the visual and emotional essence of psychedelic experiences.
- **Art Therapy:** Focuses on therapeutic and integrative aspects, using art creation to process and integrate psychedelic experiences for emotional healing and personal insight.

Guidance:

- **Psychedelic Art:** Can be created independently by the artist, without any therapeutic guidance.
- **Art Therapy:** Involves the guidance of a trained Art Therapist who helps individuals explore and process their experiences through art.

Outcome:

- **Psychedelic Art:** Aims to convey a visual representation of psychedelic experiences, often for a broad audience.
- **Art Therapy:** Aims to promote psychological healing and integration, tailored to the individual's therapeutic needs and goals.

Although psychedelic art and Art Therapy may differ, they also share many similarities that offer benefits like:

- Tapping into and activating different parts of the brain.
- Extending the liminal state of a NOSC.
- Capturing the ineffable or what words could not convey.

- Externalizing internal experience.
- Providing a form of uncensored communication.
- Connecting with the Self and Inner Healer.
- Offering rich metaphorical content for meaning-making and integration.
- Providing a way to be in dialogue with different aspects of the Self.
- Creating a meaningful thread through the phases of psychedelic experience—preparation, journey, and integration.
- Documenting the process and experience for future reference.

Psychedelic art has been a powerful medium for expressing the surreal and transcendent experiences facilitated by Psychedelics. This art form is not just about colorful, mind-bending visuals; it's about the deep, often transformative personal insights and healing that can arise from these altered states.

Notable Artists and Their Contributions

Martina Hoffmann, a contemporary of Alex Grey and a student of Stanislav Grof, creates vibrant, dream-like paintings that explore themes of feminine power, nature, and spirituality. Hoffmann's work is deeply

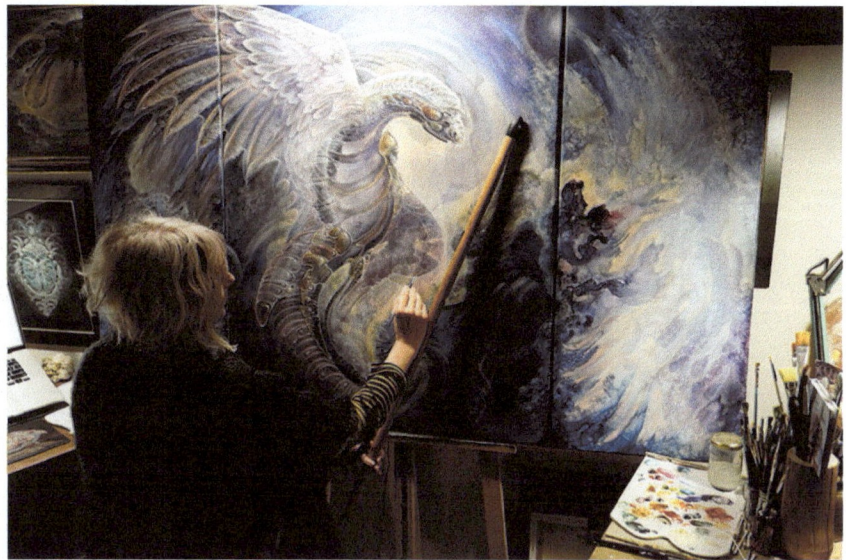

Figure 4.2 Image credit: Martina Hoffmann © in her studio painting DRAGON RIDER, 2024. www.martinahoffmann.com

influenced by her journeys with ayahuasca, a powerful entheogenic brew used traditionally in the Amazon. Her art often depicts the integration of divine feminine energy and the natural world, reflecting her own process of healing and empowerment through these profound experiences. Martina Hoffmann's work has been celebrated by many including the founder of LSD Albert Hofmann.

Alex Grey is one of the most well-known psychedelic artists. His work often depicts intricate human bodies interwoven with spiritual and mystical imagery, capturing the interconnectedness of life and the universe. Grey's art has been profoundly influenced by his own experiences with Psychedelics, particularly LSD. He describes how these substances opened his perception to the intricate, energetic structures underlying reality, which he meticulously portrays in his art. His paintings, such as "The Chapel of Sacred Mirrors," serve as a testament to the potential for art to facilitate spiritual healing and self-discovery.

Pablo Amaringo was a Peruvian artist and former shaman who is famous for his intricate, colorful depictions of ayahuasca visions. His works are a visual feast of mythical creatures, celestial beings, and vibrant plant life, each painting telling a story of his spiritual encounters. Amaringo's art provided a bridge between his Indigenous knowledge and the Western world, helping to educate and inspire many about the spiritual dimensions of ayahuasca and its healing potential.

Luis Tamani is another Peruvian artist whose work is heavily inspired by ayahuasca. His paintings are characterized by their ethereal quality and deep symbolism, reflecting the shamanic traditions and the rich biodiversity of the Amazon rainforest. Tamani's art serves as a visual narrative of his own healing journey and his connection to the natural and spiritual realms.

Allyson Grey, Alex Grey's partner, also contributes significantly to the world of psychedelic art. Her work focuses on themes of chaos, order, and secret writing, often exploring the abstract and mystical elements of consciousness. Through her art, Allyson expresses the transformative power of Psychedelics in revealing hidden dimensions of reality and the self.

As the author of this book, I felt it was relevant to include some of my own work, which has been deeply inspired by my medicinal journeys. I use art as a means of healing, transformation, and tapping into etheric realms, allowing the process of creation to become a form of channeling.

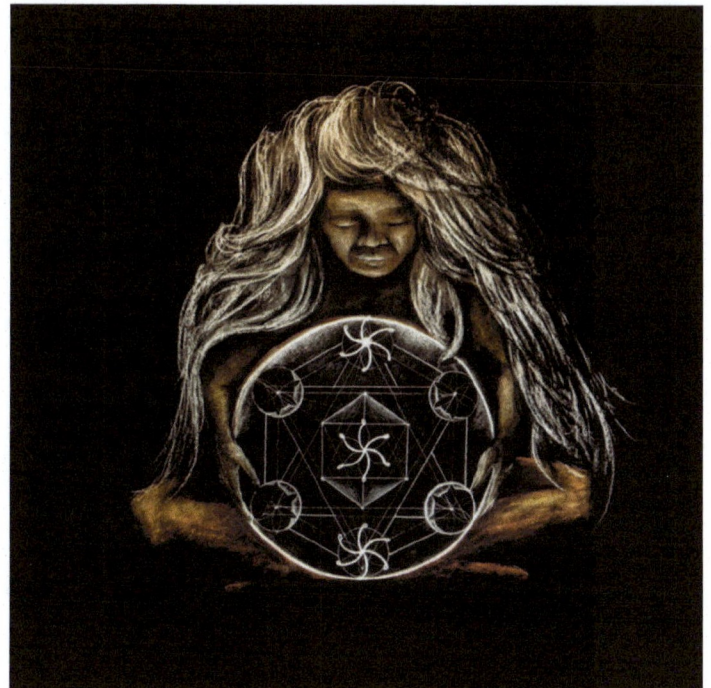

Figure 4.3 Image credit: THE MADRE SPEAKS, Charmaine Husum ©, 2019, Chalk on Black Paper. Photographed by Michael Brager

After deep meditation, my creation unfolds as I surrender to a creative force that is felt beyond my physical world. Figure 4.3 is an example of my own work, inspired by my journey with Ayahuasca. Upon reflection and meditation, it became clear to me that this woman, who I often draw, was a version of myself from another time and space. For six months she hung on my wall unfinished, where messages within the sphere she holds came forward and evolved as I continued to create.

Contribution to Healing and Integration

Psychedelic art provides a unique avenue for integrating psychedelic experiences. By translating the often ineffable and complex nature of these experiences into visual form, individuals can better understand and communicate their inner journeys. This process of externalizing internal experiences can be incredibly therapeutic, offering insights that might be difficult to access through words alone.

The act of creating psychedelic art also extends the liminal state—the threshold state of being between different phases of consciousness. This extension allows for a deeper processing of the experience, helping to ground the insights and emotions that arise during a psychedelic journey.

Art becomes a form of uncensored communication, bypassing the rational mind to tap into deeper layers of the psyche. It connects individuals with their Inner Healer, offering rich metaphorical content that aids in meaning-making and personal growth. By documenting the process and experience, individuals create a lasting record of their journey, which can be revisited for future reflection and continued healing.

The contributions of artists like Alex Grey, Martina Hoffmann, Pablo Amaringo, Luis Tamani, and Allyson Grey highlight the profound connection between art and psychedelic experiences. Their works not only capture the visual and emotional intensity of these experiences but also serve as powerful tools for integration and healing. Psychedelic art facilitates a dialogue with different aspects of the Self, helping individuals to navigate and make sense of their inner worlds. As we embrace the renaissance of Psychedelics in healing and mental health, the role of art in this process becomes increasingly vital, offering a pathway to deeper understanding and lasting transformation.

5

WHY PEOPLE SEEK ALTERED STATES

People seek altered states of consciousness for a variety of reasons, often driven by a combination of personal, psychological, and spiritual factors. These motivations include personal growth, healing, and temporary relief from life's challenges. While altered states can provide profound insights and therapeutic benefits, they also come with potential risks and should be approached with caution and respect for their power and complexity (Grof, 2000).

To Expand Consciousness and Self-Development

Many individuals are drawn to altered states as a means of exploring different aspects of consciousness and gaining deeper insights into themselves and the world around them. Such experiences can facilitate personal growth, self-discovery, and spiritual development. By transcending ordinary awareness, individuals may develop new perspectives, enhance creativity, and cultivate a deeper sense of connection with the universe (Tart, 1975). These states can dissolve the usual boundaries of the Self, leading to experiences of unity that feel transformative and healing (Wilber, 2001).

 DOI: 10.4324/9781003595762-6

To Address Trauma, Depression, and Other Mental Health Concerns

Altered states of consciousness, particularly those induced by Psychedelics or other mind-altering practices, have been recognized for their therapeutic potential in healing psychological wounds and trauma (Grof, 2000). Research has shown that these experiences can provide an opportunity to confront and process unresolved emotions and traumatic memories within a safe and supportive context (Carhart-Harris and Nutt, 2017). This process often allows for a re-framing of traumatic experiences and fosters a sense of inner peace and acceptance that traditional therapeutic methods may not achieve (Pollan, 2018).

To Escape Reality

Some individuals seek altered states to explore inner realms and expand consciousness, while others use them as a temporary escape from the pressures and stresses of daily life. These states can offer relief from anxiety, depression, and existential angst by altering perceptions and disrupting usual thought patterns (Winkelman, 2010). However, the use of altered states as a form of escapism can lead to unhealthy coping mechanisms and potential dependency on substances (Woolfe, n.d.). It is important to recognize when such use shifts from exploration to avoidance and addresses underlying issues rather than merely escaping them.

To Enhance Creativity and Problem-Solving

Altered states have been known to relax preconceived patterns of thinking, allowing individuals to make connections between seemingly unrelated ideas, thus enhancing divergent thinking (Krippner, 1994). The temporary dissolution of the internal censor during these states can lead to a free flow of novel thoughts and ideas, providing a fertile ground for creativity. This shift in consciousness may also result in hyper-associativity, where the brain connects concepts not typically linked in a standard waking state—a key aspect of creative thinking (Fadiman, 2011). Moreover, altered states can enable a different approach to problem-solving, providing perspectives not accessible in ordinary consciousness (Harman and Rheingold, 1984). For artists, writers, musicians, and other creators, such states can be a wellspring of inspiration, driving breakthroughs in their work.

To Access and Induce Spiritual or Religious Experiences

Many people seek altered states of consciousness to connect with something greater than themselves, accessing spiritual or religious experiences that provide profound personal transformation. These states can evoke a deep sense of oneness with the universe, often described as mystical experiences (James, 1902/2002). Research has shown that such experiences can lead to a re-evaluation of one's purpose in life and a deeper understanding of one's spirituality (Grof, 2000). Altered states facilitate transcendence, where the boundaries between self and the external world blur, fostering a sense of unity with all things (Tart, 1975). Many cultural and religious practices use meditation, prayer, fasting, or psychoactive substances to induce altered states, serving as integral components of rituals aimed at receiving wisdom, healing, and guidance from a higher power or one's deeper self (Eliade, 1958).

The pursuit of these experiences reflects a human longing to reconnect with the sacred and gain a more harmonious perspective on life. Whether through natural means or aided by substances, the search for spiritual experiences in altered states highlights humanity's ongoing quest for meaning, enlightenment, and a deeper sense of belonging (Wilber, 2001).

6

WAYS NON-ORDINARY STATES
ARE ACHIEVED

Psychoactive Substances

Psychoactive substances such as psilocybin, LSD (lysergic acid diethyl-amide), MDMA (3,4-Methylenedioxymethamphetamine), ayahuasca, and mescaline are widely known for their capacity to induce non-ordinary states of consciousness. Research indicates that these substances can significantly alter perception, cognition, and emotional processing, leading to unique insights, emotional healing, and spiritual experiences (Grof, 2000). Their impact on consciousness has been explored in both clinical and spiritual contexts, providing profound opportunities for self-exploration and psychological integration.

Breathwork

Techniques such as Holotropic Breathwork, developed by Stanislav Grof, involve specific breathing patterns to access altered states of consciousness. These practices can result in deep emotional release and foster a connection to one's inner experiences (Grof, 1993). Through controlled breathing, individuals may access unconscious material, promoting self-awareness and facilitating spiritual insights.

Meditation

Various meditation practices, including mindfulness, transcendental meditation, and guided visualization, can induce non-ordinary states by stilling the mind and increasing self-awareness (Walsh and Shapiro, 2006). In these states, individuals may experience altered perceptions of time, self-transcendence, and deep psychological insight. Meditation has been shown to affect brainwave patterns, fostering experiences that transcend ordinary consciousness (Tart, 1990).

Ecstatic Dance

The use of dance in spiritual and religious practices has been a method for achieving altered states across cultures. Practices such as Sufi whirling or Shamanic dancing demonstrate how physical activity can lead to spiritual and psychological transformation (Laderman and Roseman, 1996). Modern movements like 5Rhythms and ecstatic dance continue this tradition, providing a space for participants to reach a state of flow, where they become fully immersed in the rhythmic movements and their accompanying altered states of awareness (Roth, 1998).

Fasting

Fasting has been a long-standing method in many spiritual traditions to alter consciousness. By abstaining from food and drink, individuals can experience shifts in mental clarity, perception, and spiritual insight (Eliade, 1958). Fasting can alter the body's biochemical state, which, in turn, may contribute to an expanded sense of awareness and an altered relationship with the Self and the world (Cott, 1995).

Prayer

Prayer, particularly when practiced repetitively or with intense focus, can induce altered states of consciousness. Chanting, silent meditation, and other forms of prayer are known to affect brainwave activity and foster experiences of unity, peace, and connection with the divine (Newberg and Waldman, 2009). This altered state can transcend ordinary reality and facilitate profound psychological and spiritual experiences.

Ritual and Ceremony

Rituals and ceremonies have been used across cultures to induce non-ordinary states. The combination of symbolic actions, rhythmic music, chanting, and communal participation can alter consciousness and create an atmosphere conducive to personal transformation (Turner, 1969). Modern therapeutic practices continue to integrate rituals as a way to access deeper states of consciousness and facilitate healing (Eliade, 1964).

Near-Death Experiences

Near-death experiences (NDEs) occur when individuals come close to or are revived from death, often resulting in a dramatic alteration of consciousness. These experiences typically include sensations of leaving the body, encountering a transcendent light, and experiencing deep peace or interconnectedness (Ring, 1982). NDEs can catalyze significant shifts in individuals' perspectives on life, death, and the nature of consciousness (Moody, 1975).

Kundalini Awakening

Kundalini awakening, rooted in yogic traditions, involves the release of latent energy at the base of the spine, resulting in physical, emotional, and spiritual shifts (Sannella, 1987). This process can be triggered through practices such as yoga, meditation, or breathwork. The experience often includes intense sensations, vivid imagery, and a heightened state of awareness, leading to long-term changes in consciousness.

Dark Night of the Soul

The "dark night of the soul," a term popularized by the mystic St. John of the Cross, refers to a period of profound existential crisis and inner turmoil (Underhill, 1911). This state can be triggered by spiritual practices or personal challenges, pushing the individual into deep introspection and disorientation. While it is a difficult process, it can ultimately result in a transformative experience and an expanded consciousness (May, 2004).

Flow States

Flow states occur when individuals are completely absorbed in an activity, often resulting in a loss of self-consciousness and altered perception of time (Csikszentmihalyi, 1990). This state of deep engagement can lead to heightened awareness and creativity, facilitating an experience of unity and transcendent joy. Artists, musicians, and athletes frequently describe being in flow as a non-ordinary state that fosters self-expression and insight.

Additional Methods

There are other methods through which non-ordinary states of consciousness can arise. Mystical experiences, out-of-body experiences, and the use of sensory deprivation tanks have been documented as pathways to altered states (Tart, 1972). Each of these states opens new dimensions of perception and understanding, illustrating the diverse ways individuals can explore their consciousness beyond everyday reality.

7
DREAMWORK

How to Remember and Decode Your Dreams

Throughout this course, I invite you to keep an inventory of your dreams, writing them down as soon as you wake up so you are able to remember them. As you continue to collect and reflect on what is happening in your non-waking state, it will help you integrate the effects of your psychedelic experience, instilling deeper transformation and clearer awareness in your waking state (Johnson, 1986). Engaging with your dreams in this manner allows for a more conscious dialogue with your unconscious mind, fostering a sense of personal growth and self-awareness.

Paying attention to the information our dreams hold is an important component of integration and preparation. When we sleep, the unconscious and subconscious are able to fully awaken. It is in this state that deep healing can take place, as dreams provide a symbolic space where we can explore emotions and unconscious material (Hillman, 1979). This is also the arena where we can tap into etheric realms and deeper aspects of our psyche, leading to profound insights and personal transformation (Holecek, 2016). By consciously recording the information and experiences we receive upon awakening, we gain greater insight into the workings of our mind, the spirit world, and the intuitive wisdom we all hold regarding the paths that lay before us (Moss, 1996).

DOI: 10.4324/9781003595762-8

Recording our dreams is a great exercise to get used to before experiencing other non-ordinary states like Psychedelics. Even if you have already experienced a spiritual awakening, it is never too late to begin recording the images, feelings, and experiences you notice while in the dream state. This practice not only prepares you for further exploration into non-ordinary states but also helps in the ongoing process of integrating these profound experiences into daily life (Johnson, 1986; Holecek, 2016).

"I can't remember my dreams. I don't even think I dream."

This can be a common misconception, but the truth is that everyone dreams, whether they remember them or not. There are ways we can work with our inner unconscious to begin to remember our dreams. Some of my favorites include:

1. **Set an Intention before Bed**: Before going to bed, set an intention to remember your dream. You could even ask your subconscious a question you would like answered while you sleep. Write this question down to solidify your request before falling asleep.
2. **Understand Brain States**: While we sleep, we move through various brain states. In a waking state, we are at a Beta level brain state. During sleep, we move into the Alpha and Theta states, where the majority of our dreaming takes place. Alpha and Theta states are characterized as REM sleep. In this state, if we were to watch ourselves, we would notice the eyes moving from one side to another.
3. **Wake Up during REM Sleep**: To remember our dreams, it helps to wake up from these deeper sleep states. A way to do this is to drink a large glass of water before bed or set a soft alarm in the early morning hours when you are most likely in REM sleep. This will give you the opportunity to quickly record what you remember. You may be groggy upon awakening, so it is advised to use voice-to-text on your phone and vocally record what you remember from the dream. When you fall asleep again after this brief awakening, you may enter a deeper dream state, and the next time you wake up, you will be better able to recall your dream.

4. **Create a Pattern of Remembering:** As we create this pattern of remembering our experiences during our dreaming states, the information becomes more accessible, and remembering becomes part of the process. Be sure to always record the overall feeling or emotions you have after the dream, as well as whatever details you remember upon waking.

8

RECLAIMING THE ANCIENT PRACTICE OF KUNDALINI YOGA

Caveat and Important Information

Kundalini Yoga has been a part of my life since 1997, and in 2016 I became certified to teach this modality. However, like many Yogic lineages and other Guru-led exercise and meditation systems, there is a dark side that practitioners should be aware of. I urge anyone choosing to practice the techniques mentioned in this book to do so in a way that feels safe and beneficial for them (Parker, 2020).

A book published in 2020 revealed disturbing truths about the man who claimed to introduce this lineage of yoga to the West. He was found to be a sexual predator who abused numerous women and children, along with other serious transgressions (Dyson, 2020). After learning about these violations and the extensive cover-up orchestrated by the organization he founded, I stopped practicing Kundalini Yoga altogether. This was a challenging period as the practice had been central to my life. Over time, I came to recognize aspects of this lineage as cult-like (Stark and Bainbridge, 1985), and I had been fully enmeshed in its practices.

In reclaiming my practice, I researched the origins of the postures and mantras. Kundalini Yoga is an ancient practice from India, blending elements of Hatha and Raja Yoga (Feuerstein, 1998). My intention, through my own study of these ancient teachings, is to dissociate the practice

    DOI: 10.4324/9781003595762-9

from the individual who claimed to be its "inventor." This journey has empowered me and helped me move beyond a victim mentality in the wake of the deception. Knowing that he had taken so much from so many, I refused to let him take away a practice that has brought me deep healing.

I honor everyone's process when it comes to practicing this yoga. If you choose not to engage in the meditations presented here, that choice is valid. However, I have carefully selected practices that I believe are safe and disconnected from the organization that promoted the man's legacy in the West (Parker, 2020).

There are those who deny the testimonies of the brave survivors who came forward. I trust these survivors fully. If the inclusion of these yogic practices in this book upsets anyone, I apologize. It is not my intention to cause harm but rather to share aspects of Kundalini Yoga that can be credibly traced back to Indian traditions and have proven beneficial for myself and those I teach.

What Is Kundalini Yoga?

Kundalini Yoga, often referred to as the Yoga of Awareness, is accessible to people of all backgrounds and aims to rewire the brain's neurotransmitters. It works not just on the physical body but also on the nervous, endocrine, and glandular systems, supporting individuals in accessing their inner power. A major focus of the practice is the use of the drishti or eye-gaze during meditation and postures. When the eye gaze is directed between the eyebrows (third eye), pressure builds in the limbic region of the brain, activating the pituitary and pineal glands, which play a role in regulating the body's hormonal balance and mood.

Kundalini Yoga also has a unique capacity to remove emotional blocks within the body. Over time, trauma and stress can become lodged in the body, manifesting as physical ailments if not released (Levine, 2010). By bringing mindful awareness to the body and engaging in specific postures, mantras, and meditation, practitioners can invite a somatic release of these blocks, thus promoting physical and emotional healing.

The practice intentionally stresses the body when in a controlled state, helping individuals build resilience and regulate their response to stress in everyday life (Feuerstein, 1998). Techniques include eye gazes, physical movements, and mudras (hand postures) that stimulate energy pathways (nadis) in the body to achieve specific outcomes. As energy moves through the spinal column and the chakras, it creates sensations of healing, ecstasy, and peace, aligning the body and mind (Goswami, 1999).

The practice can bring up emotions as it moves and heals discordant energy stored in the body. This process is normal and invited, providing a safe space to explore and release these feelings (Levine, 2010). Practitioners are encouraged to honor their bodies and emotions, moving at their own pace. There is no expectation to push beyond what feels safe; rather, the emphasis is on connecting to one's inner wisdom to guide the process toward healing and balance.

9

THE DIFFERENCE BETWEEN AN ENTHEOGEN AND SYNTHETIC PSYCHEDELIC

Entheogens

An **entheogen** is a psychoactive substance that originates from plants or fungi and is traditionally used in spiritual or ritualistic contexts to induce altered states of consciousness and facilitate spiritual experiences. The term "entheogen" comes from the Greek words **entheos** ("full of the divine") and **genesthai** ("to become"), reflecting its sacred use in connecting with the divine or higher states of awareness (Ruck et al., 1979).

Entheogens have been employed by Indigenous cultures for thousands of years in religious ceremonies, healing practices, and rites of passage. For instance, **psilocybin mushrooms** have been used by Indigenous peoples in Central and South America for their vision-inducing properties, allowing participants to connect with spiritual entities or gain deeper insight into the self (Metzner, 2004). Similarly, **ayahuasca**, a brew made from the *Banisteriopsis caapi* vine and the *Psychotria viridis* leaf, has been used by Amazonian shamans in Peru and Brazil to facilitate healing and spiritual guidance (Shanon, 2002). **Peyote**, containing the psychoactive compound mescaline, is another well-known entheogen that has been used by Native American tribes for its mind-expanding properties during ceremonial rituals (Fikes, 1996).

These substances are not merely consumed for recreation; they are typically ingested in a ceremonial context, often guided by experienced practitioners, such as shamans or medicine people, who help facilitate the spiritual journey. The profound experiences induced by entheogens are deeply intertwined with the cultural beliefs and practices of the communities that use them (Dobkin de Rios, 1984). Because of their natural origins and historical usage in spiritual contexts, entheogens are often seen as offering a more holistic or "earth-centered" approach to exploring consciousness.

Synthetic Psychedelics

Synthetic Psychedelics, on the other hand, are laboratory-created substances that mimic or expand upon the effects of naturally occurring Psychedelics. Unlike entheogens, synthetic Psychedelics are designed through chemical processes and do not have the same direct cultural or spiritual heritage as their plant-based counterparts. The most well-known synthetic psychedelic, lysergic acid diethylamide (LSD), was first synthesized in 1938 by chemist Albert Hofmann, who later discovered its powerful mind-altering properties. Another example is 3,4-Methylenedioxyme-thamphetamine (MDMA), initially developed in 1912 by the pharmaceutical company Merck, which later gained popularity for its potential therapeutic use in psychotherapy (Sessa, 2012). 4-Bromo-2,5- dimethoxyphenethylamine (2C-B), a member of the 2C family of Psychedelics, was first synthesized in the 1970s by chemist Alexander Shulgin, known for his extensive work in creating and documenting psychoactive substances (Shulgin and Shulgin, 1991).

While synthetic Psychedelics can produce similar profound alterations in consciousness, such as enhanced sensory perception, ego dissolution, and introspective insights, they are often used in different contexts compared to entheogens. Synthetic Psychedelics have been increasingly studied in clinical settings for their potential in treating mental health conditions, including depression, anxiety, post-traumatic stress disorder (PTSD), and addiction (Carhart-Harris and Nutt, 2017). However, unlike traditional entheogenic practices, synthetic Psychedelics are usually taken without the same ceremonial or spiritual guidance, though recent therapeutic models are beginning to integrate ritualistic elements to enhance the experience (Richards, 2015).

Differences in Experience and Context

While both entheogens and synthetic Psychedelics have the potential to facilitate deep explorations of consciousness, there are notable differences in their effects, duration, and cultural contexts. **Entheogens** are often characterized by a longer, more complex interaction with the user's psyche, influenced by the natural plant's unique combination of psychoactive compounds (Tupper, 2002). For example, the ayahuasca experience involves a symbiosis of the harmala alkaloids and DMT (N,N-Dimethyltryptamine), creating a multifaceted, often visionary journey. The context of traditional use, including setting, preparation, and intention, plays a significant role in shaping the experience.

Synthetic Psychedelics, while potent in their own right, can offer a more "pure" or isolated psychoactive effect, depending on the chemical structure. The clinical use of substances like LSD and MDMA often emphasizes controlled dosages and environments, providing a safer, measurable approach to exploring altered states. However, the lack of cultural or spiritual framework around synthetic use can sometimes result in less integrated or grounded experiences unless approached with mindful intention and expert guidance (Sessa, 2012).

10

Is Ketamine a Psychedelic?

Although, ketamine is often classified as a psychedelic, it is more accurately described as a dissociative anesthetic. While it has different properties from classic Psychedelics like LSD (lysergic acid diethylamide), psilocybin, and DMT (N,N-Dimethyltryptamine), ketamine can induce profound alterations in perception, cognition, and consciousness that share similarities with psychedelic experiences.

How Ketamine Differs from Classic Psychedelics

Ketamine primarily acts on the N-methyl-D-aspartate receptors in the brain, which play a role in glutamate regulation. This is different from classic Psychedelics, which typically interact with serotonin receptors (particularly the 5-HT2A receptor). Despite this, ketamine can induce experiences that include altered sensory perception, a sense of detachment from the body (dissociation), changes in the perception of time, and deep introspective states.

Ketamine's Psychedelic Effects

Users often report that ketamine produces dream-like, out-of-body experiences and profound insights. At higher doses, it can lead to what is known as the "K-hole," a state characterized by intense dissociation

DOI: 10.4324/9781003595762-11

and vivid internal experiences that can resemble psychedelic phenomena, such as visual hallucinations, ego dissolution, and mystical-type experiences (Krystal et al., 1994).

Therapeutic Applications

Ketamine has gained attention in recent years for its therapeutic use in treating depression, PTSD, and anxiety. Ketamine-assisted psychotherapy (KAP) leverages the substance's dissociative and psychedelic-like properties to facilitate introspection, emotional processing, and therapeutic breakthroughs (Dore et al., 2019). Unlike classic Psychedelics, ketamine has a shorter duration of action, typically lasting about 1–2 hours, making it easier to manage in a clinical setting.

Classification Debate

While ketamine's primary action is as a dissociative anesthetic, it shares enough properties with Psychedelics, particularly its ability to induce non-ordinary states of consciousness and its therapeutic potential, that it is often included in discussions of Psychedelics. In fact, some researchers and clinicians refer to it as a "psychedelic-adjacent" substance or a "non-classic psychedelic" because of the nature of the experiences it can induce (Reich et al., 2022).

Is Ketamine Addictive?

While ketamine has legitimate therapeutic uses, especially in the treatment of depression and PTSD, it's addictive potential cannot be ignored. The risk of addiction is significantly higher in recreational use scenarios where the drug is used frequently, at high doses, or without medical supervision. For this reason, ketamine should be approached with caution, and its use should be monitored closely, especially in non-clinical settings.

Ketamine is currently being used legally and medically, in KAP and for its rapid-acting antidepressant effects. In clinical settings, ketamine is administered in controlled doses and under medical supervision, which minimizes the risks of addiction. The frequency of administration in therapeutic contexts (often once every few weeks) contrasts sharply with the patterns of use seen in recreational contexts, where repeated and high-dose use is more common and carries a higher risk of developing dependence.

Yes, ketamine can be addictive, though its risk profile differs from many other substances. Ketamine has the potential for both psychological dependence and, to a lesser extent, physical dependence, particularly with recreational or repeated use at high doses.

Understanding Ketamine Addiction

1. Psychological Dependence:
   - Ketamine can lead to psychological dependence, where individuals develop a strong desire to use it for its dissociative, euphoric, or mind-altering effects. The substance can provide users with temporary relief from stress, emotional pain, or reality, making it psychologically habit-forming.
   - Frequent recreational users often seek out the "K-hole" experience—a state of deep dissociation that can feel both profound and escapist. This can result in a cycle of repeated use as individuals try to re-experience those altered states.
2. Physical Dependence and Tolerance:
   - While ketamine is not known to cause significant physical withdrawal symptoms like opioids or alcohol, tolerance can develop with frequent use. Users may find that they need increasingly larger doses to achieve the desired effects, which can escalate their use.
   - Some individuals who use ketamine heavily and frequently may experience cravings and mild withdrawal symptoms, such as anxiety, depression, and agitation when they stop using it.

Risks of Long-Term or Chronic Use

Chronic ketamine use can lead to several negative health outcomes, including:

- Cognitive impairments: Long-term use has been linked to memory and cognitive deficits, which can persist even after discontinuing the drug (Morgan and Curran, 2011).

- Bladder and urinary tract issues: A well-documented consequence of chronic ketamine abuse is ketamine-induced cystitis, which can cause severe pain, frequent urination, and even bladder dysfunction (Chu et al., 2008).
- Mental health effects: Repeated use can lead to symptoms of anxiety, depression, and even psychotic-like states.

Conclusion

In summary, while ketamine is not a classic psychedelic like psilocybin or LSD, it is considered by many to be part of the broader psychedelic category due to its dissociative and mind-altering properties. Its unique mechanism of action and growing therapeutic use place it within the conversation about substances that can facilitate altered states of consciousness.

11

WHAT TO EXPECT DURING A PSYCHEDELIC JOURNEY

Each psychedelic journey is unique and can vary widely depending on a variety of factors, such as one's mindset or mood, the environment where the journey takes place, the type of psychedelic used, dosage, and any expectations one might have (Hartogsohn, 2016). The set (mindset) and setting (environment) are particularly crucial in shaping the overall experience (Zinberg, 1984).

Some common experiences you may encounter during the journey include

- **Visual Effects and Hallucinations:** Powerful and vivid visual phenomena (Shulgin and Shulgin, 1991).
- **Enhanced Sensory Perception:** Heightened awareness of sounds, sights, smells, tastes, and touch (Griffiths et al., 2008).
- **Feelings of Euphoria or Awe**: Intense joy, wonder, and a profound sense of connection (MacLean et al., 2012).
- **Ego Dissolution:** A diminished sense of self, often resulting in feelings of unity with the universe (Lebedev et al., 2015).
- **Introspection**: Deep, reflective thoughts and insights about oneself and life (Pollan, 2018).
- **Emotional Release:** Expressing and processing deep-seated emotions, sometimes long-held (Grof, 2000).

 DOI: 10.4324/9781003595762-12

- **Spiritual Insights:** Experiences that feel transcendent or mystical, often described as deeply meaningful (Griffiths et al., 2008).

Somatic responses such as nausea, restlessness, yawning, and an increased heart rate are also common occurrences during the experience (Mason et al., 2020). Emotional responses may include anxiety, panic, fear, and sadness. It's important to note that some individuals may experience nothing at all, which does not necessarily mean that the psychedelic has not had a significant effect on the brain or psyche (Carhart-Harris and Nutt, 2017).

Not all journeys are pleasant. **"Bad trips"** or challenging experiences can occur and may be characterized by:

- **Depersonalization:** Feeling detached from oneself (Lebedev et al., 2015).
- **Fear and Grief:** Intense feelings of dread or sorrow.
- **Preoccupation with Death:** Thoughts about mortality and the afterlife (Grof, 2000).
- **Paranoia and Isolation:** Distrust and feelings of being alone.
- **Panic and Physical Distress:** Extreme anxiety and discomfort (Johnson et al., 2008).

These effects are usually temporary, and with proper guidance, they are often reported as transformational opportunities, especially when explored supportively in the integration phase (Pollan, 2018).

Preparation can play a big role in shaping how the experience unfolds. This preparation might include dietary restrictions, modifying certain behaviors, and tending to one's mental and emotional state (Hartogsohn, 2016). For example, some facilitators and shamans who work with plant medicines recommend the following in preparation:

- **Avoidable Stressors:** Reducing exposure to stress whenever possible.
- **Abstinence:** Refraining from sexual activity, including with oneself.
- **Limited Screen Time:** Reducing time spent on the internet and social media.

- **Substance Avoidance:** Avoiding alcohol and recreational drugs, including marijuana.

Some traditions also suggest that the spirit of plant medicines should not be mixed with other substances in order to honor them properly (Metzner, 2004).

Again, it is important to recognize that each psychedelic journey is unique. Mindful preparation involves considering set and setting, dosage, and one's psychological state. Receiving the journey as it unfolds and, most importantly, working through what emerges during the integration phase can greatly enhance the long-term benefits of the experience (Grof, 2000).

12

PSYCHEDELIC THERAPY

THREE STAGES

Preparation

This stage can range in duration: days, weeks, or even years for some. Many who work with plant or animal medicines believe that the medicines, in fact, invite them to the psychedelic journey and experience this as a call coming through their dreams and meditations (Metzner, 2004). Maybe some of you have experienced this invitation with synthetic medicines as well?

In order to know where the messages come from (our ego, mind, the spirit of the medicine, or the energy of the experience with synthetic drugs), we need to be able to connect to the subtle energies within our bodies. By preparing for your journey through meditation, mindfulness, journaling, and the creative process, we are able to access these subtle sensations that tell us yes, no, and/or to pause and think about it. Often the messages are not clear, and that too may be a signal to continue strengthening your connection to Self (Grof, 2000). We use this building of and connection to Self throughout all stages of psychedelic therapy in this model.

Set and Setting

Set and setting refer to the psychological and environmental factors that influence the psychedelic experience. The set encompasses the

DOI: 10.4324/9781003595762-13

mindset, intentions, beliefs, and emotional state of the individual, while setting includes the physical environment in which the journey is taking place, social context, and interpersonal dynamics (Leary et al., 1963). Creating an intentionally safe, supportive set and setting is essential for promoting a positive and transformative psychedelic experience (Hartogsohn, 2016).

Preparing the Mind through Meditation Practice

Meditation practice can help individuals cultivate mindfulness, relaxation, and inner awareness, which are valuable skills for navigating the psychedelic experience. Mindfulness meditation, breathwork, and body scan exercises can help individuals develop greater presence, acceptance, and emotional regulation, enhancing their readiness for the journey (Kabat-Zinn, 2005).

For the clients I work with, I also suggest creating a routine to support:

- Control in one's life (Kabat-Zinn, 2005).
- Rerouting neural pathways (Carhart-Harris et al., 2017).
- Developing a greater appreciation and acceptance of self (Neff, 2003).
- Fostering self-esteem (Harris, 2019a).
- Connecting to something larger than themselves through a regular meditation practice (Grof, 2000).

Using Art Therapy

Art Therapy can be a valuable tool for preparing for a psychedelic journey by helping individuals access, explore, and express their intentions, fears, and hopes about the experience they are about to undertake. Art Therapy exercises such as creating mandalas, vision boards, or guided imagery can help individuals clarify their intentions, process emotions, and cultivate a sense of inner guidance and resilience (Naumburg, 1987).

You are encouraged to lean into the processes of journaling, meditation, creative exploration, becoming mindful, paying attention to your dreams, and reflecting on your intentions throughout this book.

Journey

As intense as this experience may be, it's really only a small portion of the work as far as time goes. It may last many hours, sometimes grueling, often ecstatic, but it ends, and we are left to move forward in life.

Embarking on a journey with psychedelic medicines can be a profoundly transformative experience, and the setting and guidance provided significantly influence the nature of the experience. Here are various settings in which people might engage with psychedelic substances, each offering a distinct approach and set of expectations:

Indigenous Ceremony

- **Cultural and Spiritual Context:** Indigenous shamans typically provide a deeply rooted cultural and spiritual framework for the experience. The use of Psychedelics such as ayahuasca, psilocybin, or peyote often occurs within traditional ceremonies that include rituals, prayers, and music, all intended to facilitate a spiritual journey and healing (Labate and Cavnar, 2014).
- **Environment:** These ceremonies are usually conducted in communal settings, often in nature or in dedicated ceremonial spaces, emphasizing connection to the earth and ancestral traditions (Shanon, 2002).
- **Guidance:** The shaman leads the ceremony, using their knowledge and spiritual practice to guide participants through their experiences. The shaman may intervene if they perceive that a participant is facing difficulties, using techniques passed down through generations to help navigate emotional or spiritual challenges. A shamanically guided experience is unique because the shaman is also entering into the etheric realms of the medicine and able to see and understand at a macro level what an experiencer is going through. They can intervene on these levels of spirit to enhance and facilitate deeper healing (Metzner, 2004).

Psychologist/Psychotherapist in Clinical Settings

- **Therapeutic Setting:** When psychedelic therapy is conducted by a psychologist or psychotherapist, it is usually within a controlled, clinical environment, potentially as part of a research study or therapeutic program. Common substances used include LSD (Lysergic Acid Diethylamide), MDMA (3,4-Methylenedioxyme-thamphetamine), or psilocybin (Carhart-Harris and Goodwin, 2017).

- **Safety and Monitoring:** These sessions are typically characterized by a high degree of monitoring (sometimes medical) for safety and therapeutic effectiveness. Participants are often screened for medical and psychological conditions and prepared through pre-session counseling.
- **Integration**: A psychologist or trained psychotherapist helps the participant integrate the experience and insights into their every-day life using therapeutic techniques (Johnson, 2018).

Sitter or Guide

- **Supportive Presence:** A sitter—often a trained but non-medical or non-clinical guide—provides support in more informal settings, such as a home or private retreat. Their role is primarily to ensure safety and comfort, rather than to actively guide the psy-chological journey.
- **Setting and Preparation:** The setting might be less ritualized than in Indigenous or clinical contexts, focusing instead on creating a calm, safe space. Preparation might include discussing the partici-pant's intentions and what to expect (Harris, 2019).
- **Assistance during the Experience:** Sitters generally inter-vene only to assist with practical needs or emotional support if requested, maintaining a non-intrusive presence that allows the individual's personal experience to unfold more independently (Zinberg, 1984).

Medical/Outpatient Clinic Setting with Ketamine

- **Medical Administration:** In medical settings, ketamine, origi-nally used as an anesthetic, is administered under strict medical supervision, often as a treatment for depression. This setting is highly medicalized, focusing on dosage precision, patient safety, and symptom monitoring (Dore et al., 2019).

- **Controlled Environment:** Patients receive ketamine in a tranquil, controlled clinical environment designed to promote calm and comfort during the dissociative experience that ketamine can induce.
- **Professional Oversight:** There are usually medical professionals monitoring the patient's physical and psychological responses throughout the session, providing immediate intervention if necessary.

Recreational Use: Festival and Burning Man/Raves

Festivals (like Burning Man) and cultural phenomena like Raves have their merits and challenges. They can be profoundly bonding cultural events but also expose people to the dark side of drug culture (Saunders and Doblin, 1996). Participating in such events depends on the individual's comfort with the different philosophical and cultural frameworks surrounding these experiences. Importantly, regardless of setting, it is crucial to consider the legal status of psychedelic substances in that location as well as ensure the credibility and safety standards of the organization, providers, and/or facilitators involved.

Often these events have supportive paid and volunteer staff there to support people who are having challenging experiences, such as the Zendo Project (Zendo Project, n.d.). The Fireside Project is a call center available to support people in situations where assistance is not provided, like at a rave or for individuals journeying for entertainment/diversion (Fireside Project, n.d.). Recently, many of these events are providing harm reduction safety checks to analyze medicines for hazards such as Fentanyl, but those may not always be reliable.

Role of MAPS

The Multidisciplinary Association for Psychedelic Studies (MAPS) has been instrumental in advancing the clinical research and legalization of psychedelic substances. MAPS supports rigorous studies to evaluate the therapeutic potential of Psychedelics, working closely with regulatory agencies to develop protocols that ensure safety and efficacy in treatments involving substances like MDMA for PTSD and other conditions (Doblin et al., 2019).

Integration

This is where the work really begins. The effects of altered states of consciousness can linger, bounce around, and affect our waking reality far beyond the ceremony or circumstances that brought us to that state. When our Soul's path has been opened through sacred plant medicines, entheogens, synthetic Psychedelics, or through a Kundalini awakening, dark night of the Soul, breathwork, or meditation, a profound shift occurs in the body and brain (Grof, 2000). This can be confusing when we return to our regular waking life.

Without proper integration, one might feel that further deciphering of these experiences requires more medicine, more ceremonies, or additional insights from outside of oneself. Therapeutically, this can be counterintuitive, as Trauma-informed therapy emphasizes that lasting healing comes from within (Harris, 2019). During the integration phase, one is invited to explore and deepen their relationship with the psychedelic experience itself. Integration supports the notion of connecting to and understanding one's inner self as a strength, building on this connection through reflection, creative exploration, and meditation. As this relationship grows and expands, the opportunity to create lasting changes that impact life becomes more accessible than it would be if the psychedelic experience lacked integration.

It is said that new neurons are created in the brain during a psychedelic experience (Pollan, 2018). However, it is through integration that these neural pathways become entrenched and ingrained (Carhart-Harris et al., 2017). The goal of integration is to make sense of what happened so that one feels in control of the shift presented by the non-ordinary state experience, creating a clear path toward a fulfilling, balanced, and happy life.

13

NEUROSCIENCE AND PSYCHEDELICS

How the Brain Is Affected by Non-Ordinary States

Altered states of consciousness can be profoundly moving, but what is happening in the brain to create this dramatic shift? While research on this topic is still evolving, numerous studies, functional Magnetic Resonance Imaging (fMRI) scans, and accounts from personal, professional, and medical sources help to explain the changes occurring in our brains during these deeply transformative moments (Carhart-Harris and Nutt, 2017; Griffiths et al., 2008).

One of the most powerful phenomena observed is the rerouting and creation of new neural pathways that dictate how we habitually act, react, and survive in our lives (Carhart-Harris et al., 2016). Altered states of consciousness can significantly impact these pathways, which is why they hold such potential for addressing addiction, changing detrimental habits, and transforming personality traits that may have dominated our lives.

Michael Pollan (2018) describes the mind and the pathways of neurotransmitters in the brain as being similar to a snow-covered hill where years of downhill skiing have created deep grooves. These grooves represent ingrained patterns in our lives—our habits, addictions, and the coping mechanisms we have employed to feel secure. Even when we desire to change, we often find ourselves sliding back into these established ruts, making lasting change difficult (Pollan, 2018).

DOI: 10.4324/9781003595762-14

However, a mystical or altered state experience—whether arising from meditation, a Kundalini awakening, a near-death experience, or a psychedelic ceremony—can metaphorically "level out" this snowy hill, creating a smooth surface where new pathways can be formed (Grof, 2000). This resurfacing of the brain is part of the neuroscience behind mystical and entheogenic experiences; the brain is given an opportunity to restructure itself, facilitating changes in behavior and potentially allowing a new life to emerge (Carhart-Harris et al., 2017).

As transformational as these experiences can be, there is a risk of becoming overly reliant on them. Sometimes, the pursuit of altered states can become its own rut in the snow. One might find themselves constantly seeking these dramatic shifts—spending hours in meditation, increasing intake or dosage of Psychedelics like psilocybin, LSD, or ayahuasca, jumping from one healing retreat to another, or constantly searching for the next guru (Pollan, 2018). This repeated seeking outside of oneself can become an obstacle, distracting from the true goal: healing and growth from within.

The goal is to foster internal healing so that the desired changes in life are lasting. As Harris (2019) points out, lasting healing comes from within, rather than relying on external sources. This book focuses on the empowerment that arises when our healing originates from within, allowing us to actively reshape our neural pathways for enduring effects.

The protocols outlined in this book were created to support this process. Through integration, we can maintain these new ways of being beyond the initial experience, applying the changes to our everyday lives. This approach allows the newly formed neural pathways to support our continued evolution, healing, and personal growth. Integration sustains our greatness and helps us stop seeking outside ourselves for what already resides within. This is my hope for all those on the path of transformation, to fully experience the power of neuroplasticity and that we can change our minds.

Optimizing Brain Function with Art and Meditation

Art Therapy and meditation share the powerful healing effect of integrating the left and right hemispheres of the brain. Typically, the left hemisphere is associated with orderly, statistical, mathematical, logical, and rational thinking—it processes information in a linear manner (Gazzaniga, 2000). In contrast, the right hemisphere represents passion, sensory experiences, creativity, free-spiritedness, imagination, and the vividness of colors and emotions (McGilchrist, 2012).

Without activities that stimulate integration between both sides of the brain, it becomes challenging for one hemisphere to make sense of how the other perceives the world. For example, feelings and expressions cannot simply be put into the "boxes" that the left hemisphere prefers; they need to be experienced fully to be understood. Conversely, the right hemisphere may struggle to comprehend the structured and analytical processes of the left brain. As a society, we often prioritize left-brain dominance, which can create an imbalance, disrupting the natural flow of daily living (Iacoboni, 2009). This is why creating integration and balance within both sides of the brain is so essential.

Observing, drawing, or creating art fosters this integration in a deeply therapeutic manner (Malchiodi, 2015). Similarly, meditation, mindfulness practices, and various yogic postures help to harmonize the hemispheres of the brain. Whenever we engage in activities that require both logical and creative thought, we support the integration of the brain's hemispheres.

Both meditation and Art Therapy facilitate changes in the brain by rerouting neurotransmitters and reshaping neural pathways. As neuropsychologist Donald Hebb famously stated, "Neurons that fire together, wire together," highlighting how repeated experiences strengthen connections in the brain (Hebb, 1949). This principle explains how our habits and patterns of behavior are formed—some of which may limit our potential. Through mindful awareness of emotions, bodily sensations, and creative expression, Art Therapy and meditation provide powerful tools for exploring new ways of being. By engaging with these practices, individuals can break free from limiting patterns and cultivate greater self-awareness. When integrated into psychedelic therapy, these approaches deepen the connection to one's inner resources, fostering transformative growth and personal empowerment.

What Is Happening in the Brain?

When someone uses Psychedelics, their brain undergoes several significant changes that affect perception, emotion, and cognition. Here's a breakdown of what typically happens:

1. **Serotonin Receptor Agonism:** Most classic Psychedelics, such as LSD, psilocybin, and DMT, function primarily by acting as agonists of serotonin receptors, particularly the 5-HT2A receptor (Nichols, 2016). This means they bind to these receptors and activate them, mimicking the effects of serotonin, a neurotransmitter associated with feelings of well-being and happiness. The activation of these receptors is thought to lead to the perceptual changes that occur during a psychedelic experience, including visual hallucinations and altered thought processes.

2. **Increased Brain Connectivity:** Brain imaging studies have shown that Psychedelics significantly increase connectivity across different regions of the brain (Petri et al., 2014). Normally, brain activity tends to be relatively segregated, with different tasks or functions handled by specific networks. Under the influence of Psychedelics, these networks break down, forming new connections and leading to more integrated and novel patterns of communication across the brain. This can manifest as synesthesia (e.g., "seeing" sounds or "hearing" colors), profound shifts in perspective, or feelings of interconnectedness with the universe (Carhart-Harris et al., 2014).

3. **Decreased Default Mode Network (DMN) Activity:** The DMN is a network of brain regions typically active during rest and involved in self-referential thoughts and feelings (Raichle, 2015). Psychedelics have been found to reduce activity in the DMN, which some researchers connect with the experience of ego dissolution that is often reported during psychedelic experiences (Carhart-Harris et al., 2012). This decrease in DMN activity may also explain why Psychedelics can be effective in treating conditions like depression, where overactivity of the DMN is commonly observed (Sheline et al., 2019).

4. **Emotional Amplification and Release:** Psychedelics can amplify emotional states, making users more sensitive to their environments (Grof, 2000). This amplification can lead to intense emotional experiences, both positive and negative. Importantly, this emotional amplification can have therapeutic outcomes, as individuals confront and process emotions or memories they may have previously suppressed.

5. **Therapeutic Effects:** Beyond the acute effects of a psychedelic experience, long-term changes in mood, attitudes, and behaviors have been reported and studied clinically. Psychedelic therapies have shown promising results for conditions like depression, PTSD, and addiction, often attributed to the substances' ability to induce profound, meaningful experiences that foster personal insight and psychological growth (Griffiths et al., 2016).

These effects, while potentially beneficial, also carry risks. The experience can vary widely based on the individual's mindset (set) and environment (setting), as well as the specific substance and dosage used (Hartogsohn, 2016).

What Is the Default Mode Network?

The DMN is a set of interacting brain structures first described in 2001 by neuroscientist Marcus Raichle (Raichle et al., 2001). It is most active when the brain is in a resting state, which is why it is referred to as the "default mode." This network links parts of the cerebral cortex (involved in thinking, decision-making, and other higher brain functions) with deeper, evolutionarily older brain structures responsible for emotion and memory.

The DMN is said to influence and often inhibit other parts of the brain, particularly those involved in emotion and memory, preventing signals from interrupting or interfering with each other. Neuroimaging studies suggest that the DMN plays a role in higher-order "metacognitive" activities such as self-reflection, mental projection, time travel (i.e., thinking about the future or past), and the ability to attribute mental states to others (Sheline et al., 2019).

What is particularly interesting is the connection between DMN and the ego. The DMN is believed to house the part of our brain responsible for judgment, tolerance, reality testing, and a sense of self—what Freud referred to as the "ego" (Freud, 1923). Michael Pollan (2018) describes this area of the brain as the "me" network. When individuals are asked to consider adjectives related to their self-identity, this network lights up. It also becomes active during daydreams, magical thinking, self-reflection, and even when receiving social media validation, like Facebook likes (Pollan, 2018). Therefore, when the brain is not focused on a particular task, the DMN activates "by default."

Freud posited that the ego keeps the anarchic forces of the id in check, and Pollan compares this function to the DMN's regulation of strict neural connections formed throughout adult life. "It appears that when activity in the DMN falls off precipitously, the ego temporarily vanishes, and the usual boundaries we experience between self and world, subject and object, all melt away," Pollan stated (2018).

Being able to notice when we are acting from a place of ego, instead of from mindful awareness, can profoundly change how we interact with the world. This concept is sometimes referred to as "getting out of your own way" to allow your destiny or Dharmic path to unfold. As British philosopher Alan Watts eloquently put it, "Ego, the self which he has believed himself to be, is nothing but a pattern of habits" (Watts, 1966). Mindfulness and Art Therapy help us cultivate new habits and awareness that embrace the world around us rather than focusing solely on ourselves.

Mindfulness Definition

Paying attention to the present moment, on purpose, nonjudgmentally.

(Jon Kabat-Zinn, 1994)

Current research reveals that the internal chatter—often referred to as "monkey mind" in Buddhist practice—that leads our thoughts astray during meditation is actually the DMN in action. It becomes engaged when the brain is unoccupied (Brewer et al., 2011). Through mindfulness and meditation, we can quiet this monkey mind chatter, effectively turning off the DMN to bring about a greater sense of calm and peacefulness. Additionally, being in a state of mindfulness helps keep the frontal lobes online, allowing us to integrate experiences and emotions rather than dissociate from them (Ogden, 2019).

When we experience stress, the prefrontal cortex can go offline, impairing our judgment. "Mindfulness keeps the frontal lobes online and helps integrate rather than dissociate," as noted by Ogden (2019). Engaging with the body by observing physical sensations and their transient nature can be an effective practice. By noticing that our physical sensations are not permanent, we become aware that our current state of being is changeable, offering hope when life's stresses feel overwhelming.

Dissociation is also associated with altered activity in the Default Mode Network (DMN), reflecting disruptions in self-referential thinking and emotional processing. While dissociation can serve as a defense mechanism during overwhelming experiences, personal growth involves creating new habits and neural pathways that help us move beyond outdated coping strategies, fostering greater alignment with our highest consciousness.

Research has found a significant correlation between DMN and conditions like depression and anxiety. Studies show that individuals experiencing these conditions often have more activity in the DMN areas of the brain (Marwood and Wise, 2017). "The baseline imaging findings are consistent with those found in patients with major depressive disorder and suggest that increased connectivity within the DMN may be important in the pathophysiology of both acute and chronic manifestations of depressive illness" (Posner et al., 2013). When we practice mindfulness and return to the present moment, we can interrupt the cycle of rumination that exacerbates feelings of depression and anxiety (Scott-Alexander, 2023). Mindfulness can literally make us happier—a valuable tool to keep close.

In Art Therapy, we work to reroute neural networks to change patterns, habits, and behaviors. If the DMN activates, it can inhibit this change. As neuroscientist and author Dan Siegel states, "Your mind can change your molecules" (Siegel, 2010a). Therefore, staying present and recognizing when we go "offline" is crucial. Learning anything new is a process, so be gentle with yourself. The more you practice coming back to the present moment, the more ingrained these new neural pathways become.

May you find grace on your journey toward mindful awareness and keeping your DMN from clouding your ability to remain present and happy.

The Similarities between Art, Meditation, and Psychedelics

Making Art:

- **Neural Activation:** Brain scans of individuals engaged in artistic creation often show activity in the frontal lobe, which is associated with higher cognitive functions such as decision-making, problem-solving, and planning (Bolwerk et al., 2014). The parietal lobe, responsible for processing sensory information, also becomes active during artistic activities, aiding in the translation of vision into motor coordination.
- **DMN Activity:** Artistic activities tend to decrease activity in the DMN, indicating a shift away from self-referential thoughts toward a more task-focused state (Beaty et al., 2015). Artists frequently describe being "in the zone," or entering a flow state where they lose track of time and self, which aligns with this DMN suppression.

Meditation:

- **Neural Effects:** During meditation, especially forms focused on mindfulness or concentrated attention, there is typically increased activity in the prefrontal cortex and decreased activity in the DMN (Brewer et al., 2011). This reduction is associated with a decrease in mind-wandering and a greater focus on the present moment.
- **Different Meditation Styles:** Various meditation styles may affect the DMN differently. For example, open-monitoring meditation (such as Zen) can lead to unique integration within the network, promoting a broad, non-attached awareness of thoughts and sensations (Garrison et al., 2015).

Using Psychedelics:

- **DMN Suppression:** Psychedelic substances like psilocybin or LSD often result in decreased DMN activity, correlating with users reporting feelings of ego dissolution or a diminished sense of self (Carhart-Harris et al., 2012). This effect is coupled with increased connectivity across different brain regions, contributing to the heightened sense of connectedness and unusual sensory perceptions noted during psychedelic experiences.
- **Enhanced Brain Interconnectivity:** The suppression of DMN activity under Psychedelics and the concurrent increase in brain interconnectivity might explain the profound changes in perception, thought, and emotion associated with these substances (Carhart-Harris et al., 2014).

Correlation between Activities and the DMN

All three activities—making art, meditation, and using Psychedelics—involve altering the brain's usual state of activity, particularly affecting the DMN. The DMN serves as a cognitive baseline or autopilot, engaging during routine, self-focused thoughts and disengaging when attention is directed outward or the mind experiences significant alteration (Raichle, 2015). Understanding these shifts helps explain how various activities impact mental states and consciousness, providing insights that can potentially be harnessed for therapeutic benefits. Each activity, whether through suppression or integration of the DMN, highlights different aspects of how the brain manages focus, self-awareness, and external engagement.

Ego Dissolution

Ego dissolution, often reported in the context of psychedelic experiences, refers to a profound alteration in self-perception where the boundaries that typically define and separate one's sense of self from the external world and others become blurred or even disappear entirely (Nour et al., 2016).

In practical terms, during ego dissolution, individuals might experience a loss of the usual mental filters and defenses, leading to a sense of unity and interconnectedness with the universe, other people, and nature (Lebedev et al., 2015). This phenomenon can manifest as feeling as though one is merging with their surroundings or losing the typical sense of being a distinct individual. The experience may be accompanied by a deep sense of oneness or a feeling of transcendence beyond the self.

The implications of ego dissolution in psychedelic therapy are significant. By temporarily reducing the dominance of the ego, Psychedelics can help individuals break free from rigid patterns of thought and behavior. This state can provide therapeutic benefits, particularly for conditions marked by excessive self-focus and rigid thinking, such as depression, anxiety, and PTSD (Carhart-Harris et al., 2018a). The experience can lead to insights and emotional releases that are often difficult to access through traditional therapy alone.

From a therapeutic perspective, the experience of ego dissolution may facilitate a deeper exploration of one's thoughts and feelings without the usual defensive mechanisms. This open state allows individuals to confront and integrate aspects of the self that they might be unaware of or actively avoid in everyday consciousness, potentially leading to transformative psychological healing and growth (Watts et al., 2017). The dissolution of ego boundaries can promote a more flexible mindset and foster a sense of interconnectedness, which can be a catalyst for lasting positive change.

14

INDIGENOUS PERSPECTIVES ON HEALING AND MEDICINAL PLANT SPIRITS

Indigenous cultures have developed a profound knowledge of psycho-active plants through a combination of deep environmental connections and extensive observation of their natural surroundings. This knowledge often stems from a long history of trial-and-error experimentation and keen observation of the effects of these plants on both humans and animals. For example, witnessing animals consuming certain plants and then exhibiting altered behavior could lead a shaman to explore the plant's potential for human use (Schultes and Hofmann, 1980).

Many Indigenous traditions hold that the discovery and use of psychedelic plants were revealed through spiritual means. These revelations often occur during dreams, visions, or through direct communication with the plant's spirit (Tafur, 2017). Such experiences are deeply embedded in the cultural fabric and are passed down through myths, stories, and oral traditions (Luna, 1984b). In these cultures, plants are seen not merely as tools or medicines but as conscious entities with their own spirits, guiding humans toward healing and knowledge.

The exchange of knowledge between different tribes and communities through migration and trade routes also played a significant role in the spread of the use of psychedelic plants. As various groups interacted, they shared not only goods but also medicinal practices, including the use of Psychedelics (Dobkin de Rios, 1984). This exchange enriched the

DOI: 10.4324/9781003595762-15

collective understanding of plant medicine and the diverse ways in which it could be integrated into spiritual and communal practices.

Psychedelics found their way into the core of spiritual and ceremonial practices for several distinct reasons:

- **Spiritual Insights**: They provided a means to gain spiritual insights and connect with divine entities, ancestors, or spirits (Fotiou, 2020).
- **Rites of Passage**: Psychedelics served as essential elements in rites of passage, marking critical transitions in an individual's life, such as puberty, marriage, or entry into adulthood (Eliade, 1958).
- **Healing**: These plants were employed for healing, seen as medicines capable of treating physical, psychological, and spiritual maladies. In many Indigenous cultures, healers or shamans use these substances to diagnose and cure illnesses, often facilitated by entering a trance or altered state of consciousness (Dobkin de Rios and Janiger, 2003).
- **Community Cohesion**: The communal psychedelic experience enhanced social bonds and mutual understanding, often fostering a sense of unity and collective purpose (Tupper, 2002).
- **Divination**: They were used for divination, offering guidance and answers to significant communal questions, assisting in decision-making for the community or individuals (Harner, 1980).

The incorporation of Psychedelics into ceremonies is motivated by more than the pursuit of their psychoactive effects; it represents a conduit to deeper spiritual understanding. These substances are regarded as sacred, and their use is often surrounded by ritual and respect, reinforcing the cultural values and beliefs central to the community's way of life (Labate and Cavnar, 2014). In Indigenous contexts, the use of these medicines is not a recreational activity but a deeply spiritual practice, one that requires preparation, intention, and a sense of reverence for the plant spirits involved.

Traditional Use and Rituals

Indigenous shamans have used psychoactive substances for centuries as a means to bridge the physical and spiritual worlds, accessing insights, healing, and guidance. This use of plant medicines is not merely a matter of consumption; it involves elaborate rituals and a deep understanding of the substances' spiritual significance. Here are some commonly used substances and their associated traditions:

Ayahuasca

Used predominantly in the Amazon Basin, ayahuasca is a brew made from the *Banisteriopsis caapi* vine and other plant ingredients containing the psychoactive compound DMT. The ceremonial use of ayahuasca by Amazonian tribes, such as the Shipibo and the Ashaninka, involves extensive preparation rituals led by a shaman (Curandero). The ceremony often includes chanting and the singing of Icaros—sacred healing songs believed to guide participants through their visions and assist in their spiritual journey (Labate and Cavnar, 2014). Group participation is integral, as the collective experience fosters a sense of community and shared transformation.

Peyote

Peyote has been an important sacrament for many Native American tribes, especially those in North America. In the Native American Church, peyote ceremonies involve prayer, singing, and contemplation. These ceremonies are typically performed in a circle, often lasting overnight, and are facilitated by a designated "Roadman" who leads the participants through the ritual (Stewart, 1987). The use of peyote is seen as a way to connect with spiritual guides, gain insights, and promote personal healing. The rituals are deeply rooted in the cultural and religious practices of the tribes, emphasizing respect for the plant as a sacred medicine.

Psilocybin Mushrooms

Indigenous groups in Mesoamerica, such as the Mazatec people of Mexico, have long used psilocybin mushrooms in their spiritual practices. These ceremonies are often conducted by a shaman or curandero who provides direct guidance to participants, helping them navigate the visions and emotions that arise during the experience. Ritual elements include prayer, chanting, and the use of sacred objects to create an environment conducive to healing and insight (Wasson, 1980). The mushroom's effects are considered a doorway to the spiritual realm, facilitating communication with divine entities or ancestral spirits.

These traditional uses are not focused solely on the psychoactive effects of the substances but rather on their ability to facilitate spiritual exploration and healing. The role of the shaman or guide in these ceremonies is crucial, as they possess the knowledge and skills to create a safe and sacred space for participants to undergo their transformative experiences. The integration of these substances into cultural and religious rituals underscores their importance in Indigenous worldviews, which see the physical and spiritual as interconnected aspects of existence.

Evolution over the Years

Over the years, traditional practices involving psychoactive substances have evolved due to various influencing factors:

- **Cultural Exchange**: With increased globalization, cultural exchanges have introduced these practices to a wider audience. This exposure has sometimes led to the adaptation of rituals to fit new contexts or make them more accessible to non-Indigenous participants (Fotiou, 2020). While some view this as an opportunity for cross-cultural learning and spiritual growth, others express concern about the potential for cultural appropriation and the loss of ritual authenticity (Graveline, 1998).
- **Legal and Political Pressures**: Indigenous communities have often encountered legal and political obstacles in maintaining their traditional practices. The use of psychoactive substances like ayahuasca and peyote has been scrutinized at both national and international levels, resulting in regulatory challenges. However, efforts to legalize or decriminalize these substances in some regions have led to changes in how and where these ceremonies are conducted (Labate and Feeney, 2012). For example, in places where Psychedelics are becoming legalized, practitioners are adapting their ceremonies to fit within a more structured, clinical environment.
- **Tourism and Commercialization**: The growing interest in psychedelic tourism has influenced how some Indigenous communities conduct their ceremonies. While the influx of visitors has

provided an economic boost, it has also led to the commercialization of sacred rituals, raising concerns about cultural sensitivity, commodification, and the risk of exploitation (George et al., 2020). The spiritual essence of these practices can be diluted when they are offered as a commodity rather than as a sacred, transformative experience.

- **Environmental Changes**: Climate change, deforestation, and agricultural expansion have impacted the natural environments where psychoactive plants like *Banisteriopsis caapi* (used in ayahuasca) and peyote grow. These changes affect the availability of crucial ingredients, altering traditional harvesting methods and sometimes limiting access to these sacred plants (Labate and Cavnar, 2014). The scarcity of these natural resources has sparked conversations about sustainability and the importance of preserving the ecosystems that support these sacred plants.
- **Technological Integration**: The modern era has brought technological integration into these practices. The recording and sharing of ceremonies via digital media have helped preserve some aspects of traditional rituals, allowing knowledge to be passed on to future generations. However, this practice raises questions about privacy and the sanctity of these traditions. For many Indigenous communities, the ceremonies are sacred experiences meant to be kept within the confines of their culture, not to be broadcast or commercialized (Tupper, 2002).

Despite these changes, many Indigenous communities strive to preserve the integrity and authenticity of their psychoactive medicinal practices. They emphasize the importance of respect, tradition, and spirituality, urging participants to approach these experiences with reverence and a genuine desire for personal and spiritual growth (Smith, 2000). This commitment to preserving cultural heritage amidst evolving external pressures reflects the resilience and adaptability of these ancient practices (Wilson, 2008).

What Is a Shaman?

A shaman is a figure often found in various Indigenous cultures around the world, recognized for their ability to act as intermediaries or communicators between the human world and the spirit worlds (Eliade, 1964). Shamans are usually healers, spiritual leaders, and visionaries who play a central role in their communities by managing, interpreting, and mediating the spiritual aspects of life (Graveline, 1998; Walsh, 2007). Here are some key aspects of the role of a shaman:

- **Spiritual Mediator:** Shamans are believed to have the ability to enter altered states of consciousness at will, allowing them to communicate with spirits, engage with spiritual dimensions, and travel to spiritual realms. This unique capability enables them to gain insights, seek guidance, and request help from spirit entities (Harner, 1990).
- **Healer:** One of the primary roles of a shaman is that of a healer (Graveline, 1998). They use a variety of tools and techniques, including herbal medicine, rituals, music, and dance, to treat physical, emotional, mental, and spiritual ailments. Their healing practices are often based on the belief that illness is caused by spiritual imbalances or disruptions (Kleinman, 1980).
- **Ritual Specialist:** Shamans conduct various ceremonial activities intended to influence the spiritual world for the benefit of the community or individual. This might include rituals for healing, fertility, rainmaking, or warding off evil spirits (Lévi-Strauss, 1963).
- **Custodian of Myth and Lore:** Shamans often hold a vast knowledge of cultural traditions, myths, songs, and histories of their people. They are responsible for passing this knowledge on to future generations, thus preserving cultural heritage (Tedlock, 2005).
- **Psychopomp:** In many traditions, shamans also act as "psychopomps," guiding the spirits of the deceased to the afterlife. This role underscores the shaman's ability to navigate between different worlds (Eliade, 1964).
- **Seer and Diviner:** Shamans frequently perform divinations to predict future events or uncover hidden knowledge. This aspect of their role helps the community make informed decisions about forthcoming actions (Harner, 1990).

The training to become a shaman is often rigorous, involving long periods of apprenticeship and numerous trials to master the spiritual, medicinal, and ritual knowledge required for the role (Walsh, 2007). This apprenticeship is sometimes prompted by a spiritual calling, marked by specific dreams, visions, or near-death experiences, which are seen as signs of selection by the spirits.

Shamanism, in its various forms, is practiced across the globe, from the shamans of Siberia and the Amazonian ayahuasqueros to the healers in sub-Saharan Africa. Each culture adapts the role to its specific spiritual and community needs, making shamanism a diverse and complex global phenomenon (Lévi-Strauss, 1963).

How Are We Able to Honor the Title of Shaman in Western Cultures?

The debate over whether it's culturally appropriate for non-Indigenous individuals to call themselves "shamans" raises several complex issues around cultural sensitivity, appropriation, and respect for Indigenous traditions (Kirmayer, 2004). Indigenous communities often view the term "shaman" as deeply entwined with their cultural and spiritual practices (Graveline, 1998). When non-Indigenous people adopt this title without a legitimate lineage or deep, sustained engagement with these communities, it can constitute cultural appropriation (Smith, 2012). Taking from another culture without a true understanding or respect for its significance is especially troubling given the historical context of colonialism, where appropriating and diluting the cultures of marginalized groups has been commonplace (Simpson, 2017).

The misuse of the term can also dilute its original meaning and strip it of its profound cultural and spiritual significance, transforming a role steeped in responsibility and traditional knowledge into a vacuous label designed for commercial gain (Znamenski, 2007). This commercialization is particularly exploitative when the profits of these pseudo-spiritual practices are not reciprocally shared with the Indigenous groups from which they came (Wallace, 2003).

While some argue that non-Indigenous individuals who have been trained by an Indigenous shaman and recognized by that community may have the right to use the title, this should only be done with explicit consent and appropriate acknowledgment of their training's origins (Walsh, 2007). Moreover, it is advisable for non-Indigenous practitioners to adopt alternative terms such as "spiritual healer" or "energy worker" that do not carry the same cultural weight and potential for misappropriation as "shaman" (Harner, 1990).

Non-Indigenous individuals interested in shamanistic practices must take on the responsibility to educate themselves about the cultural, historical, and spiritual backgrounds of these practices (Kirmayer, 2004). Engaging with them respectfully, informatively, and with an awareness of their origins is crucial. This includes using alternative designations and engaging in continuous respectful dialogue and learning about the traditions they explore (Smith, 2012).

In summary, the interest in shamanistic practices can be a part of a genuine spiritual search or therapeutic pursuit. However, it is essential for non-Indigenous people to approach these traditions with humility and respect, fully aware of the broader cultural implications of adopting such a title as "shaman." This approach helps honor and participate in these spiritual practices in a way that honors and preserves the integrity of the cultures that have nurtured them (Simpson, 2017).

Bruja Energy—What Is It?

(Trigger Warning—some content may upset readers)

In some cultural contexts, the concept of "bruja energy" is associated with malevolent forces and can be seen as akin to sorcery or black magic (Gordon, 2018). This negative aspect of bruja energy is distinctly characterized by its harmful intentions and disruptive influence, particularly within Indigenous ceremonies that involve the use of plant medicines. Unlike the positive aspects of the term "bruja," which focuses on healing and empowerment, this negative application deals with the intentional use of spiritual knowledge to cause harm or chaos (Anzaldúa, 1987).

This form of bruja energy might manifest as an external, intrusive force during spiritual or healing ceremonies, where it is specifically directed to interfere with the positive and restorative intentions of a shaman or the participating group (Metzner, 1999). The objective can range from causing general disruption to inflicting direct harm on individuals, thereby corrupting the sacred and therapeutic aspects of the ceremony.

Within many Indigenous shamanic traditions, there is a significant emphasis on spiritual warfare, which involves defending against and countering such malevolent practices (Eliade, 1964). Practitioners who are knowledgeable in the use of plant medicines might employ various strategies to combat this negative energy. This includes the use of specific herbs known for their protective qualities, which may be burned or used to create barriers against spiritual attacks (Harner, 1990). Additionally, rituals might be conducted to cleanse the affected individuals or spaces, thereby restoring harmony and protection.

Plant medicines also play a crucial role in healing the spiritual damage inflicted by such attacks. Certain herbs and concoctions are valued not just for their physical healing properties but also for their ability to restore spiritual well-being (Beyer, 2009). In cases where negative bruja energy has left a mark, these plant-based treatments are integral to the healing ceremonies that aim to cleanse, heal, and protect the community or individuals.

Furthermore, some plant medicines are believed to possess the power to directly counteract sorcery or black magic (Dobkin de Rios, 1984). These plants can be used in more aggressive forms of spiritual countermeasures, effectively reversing curses or neutralizing harmful spells. This use of plant medicines highlights their dual nature in Indigenous spiritual practices—not only as agents of healing and enlightenment but also as tools for spiritual defense and restoration (Mabit, 2007).

Thus, the concept of bruja energy, when viewed as a negative force, encompasses the misuse of spiritual power for harmful ends, standing in stark contrast to the beneficial uses of plant medicines in Indigenous ceremonies. The practitioners' deep knowledge of both the healing and protective properties of plants is crucial in maintaining the balance and safety of their spiritual and communal practices (Gordon, 2018).

The Importance of Creating a Sacred Circle

In Ayahuasca ceremonies, where the spiritual openness and vulnerability of participants can be heightened, Indigenous shamans implement various protective measures to safeguard against negative energies (Dobkin de Rios and Rumrrill, 2008). These practices are deeply rooted in shamanic tradition and are vital to ensuring the safety and integrity of the healing experience. Here are some examples of practices shamans might use during Ayahuasca ceremonies to guard against such negative influences:

1. **Setting a Sacred Space:** Shamans begin by creating a sacred space, often through the ritualistic clearing and blessing of the area where the ceremony will take place (Luna, 1984b). This might involve the use of smoke from sacred herbs like palo santo, sage, or tobacco (Graveline, 1998). The smoke is believed to purify the space from negative energies and establish a protective barrier (Harner, 1990).

2. **Invocations and Prayers:** At the start of the ceremony, shamans invoke the protection of spiritual entities or forces. These might include ancestral spirits, nature spirits, or other protective deities associated with their cultural practices (Luna and Amaringo, 1999). Through prayers and chants, they ask for safety, guidance, and clarity for all participants.

3. **Use of Protective Talismans or Amulets**: Participants may be given talismans or amulets to wear during the ceremony. These items are often blessed by the shaman and are believed to carry protective powers. They can include stones, crystals, beads, or small bags containing sacred herbs or relics (Metzner, 1999).

4. **Ritual Offerings:** Shamans often make offerings to the spirits as a way of ensuring their favor and protection during the ceremony. These offerings can include food, libations, or other items considered valuable or sacred within the culture (Beyer, 2009).

5. **Icaros or Sacred Songs:** Throughout the Ayahuasca ceremony, shamans sing Icaros, traditional healing songs believed to direct the spiritual and healing journey of the ceremony (Dobkin de Rios and Rumrrill, 2008). Icaros are also used to ward off negative spirits and energies, guide the participants through their visions, and invoke protective spirits.

6. **Spiritual Cleansing Before and After:** Shamans may perform individual cleansings on participants using sacred herbs, feathers, or hands-on energy work before and after consuming Ayahuasca (Luna, 1984b). These cleansings help to remove negative energy that participants might bring into the space or accumulate during the ceremony.

7. **Constant Vigilance and Adaptation:** During the ceremony, the shaman remains alert to the energies and dynamics of the group (Harner, 1990). If they sense any negative energy or spiritual disturbance, they can modify their chants, focus their healing efforts on specific individuals, or perform additional rituals to restore harmony and protection to the group.

8. **Closing Ritual:** At the end of the ceremony, a closing ritual is performed to thank the protective spirits, seal off the sacred space from any lingering negative energies, and ensure that participants are grounded and cleared before they leave (Beyer, 2009).

These protective practices are integral to the safety and effectiveness of Ayahuasca ceremonies. They reflect a deep understanding of the spiritual dimensions involved in these rituals and demonstrate the shaman's role not only as a guide to altered states of consciousness but also as a guardian against spiritual harm (Luna and Amaringo, 1999).

The Impact of Sacred Songs

Icaros are traditional healing songs or chants used by Indigenous shamans, particularly in the Amazon basin, during ceremonies involving psychedelic medicines like Ayahuasca (Luna, 1984a). These songs are considered one of the most vital and powerful tools in shamanic practice. Their use in ceremonies is deeply interwoven with the belief systems and therapeutic processes of Indigenous cultures (Beyer, 2009). Here's a deeper look into how Icaros are used and their significance compared to ceremonies involving other psychedelic substances where such elements may not be utilized.

Usage of Icaros in Ceremonies

- **Guiding the Experience:** Shamans sing specific Icaros to invoke the spirit of Ayahuasca, to call upon other spiritual entities for protection and assistance, and to manage the intensity and nature of the participants' experiences (Dobkin de Rios and Rumrrill, 2008). These Icaros help navigate the visionary states, enhancing the therapeutic and revelatory aspects of the journey. The melodies and rhythms of the Icaros can modulate the participants' emotional and spiritual experiences, steering them toward insight, healing, and transformation (Luna and Amaringo, 1999).

• **Protection Against Negative Energies**: Icaros are also used to protect the ceremonial space and the participants from negative energies and spiritual entities (Mabit, 2007). The shaman chants these protective Icaros to create a safe healing environment, ensuring that the space remains consecrated and guarded throughout the session. This protective aspect of Icaros is crucial, as participants in Ayahuasca ceremonies are often in vulnerable and heightened states of consciousness that can make them more susceptible to spiritual intrusions (Beyer, 2009).

The use of Icaros contrasts significantly with other psychedelic ceremonies where such elements may not be present, highlighting the distinct cultural and spiritual contexts of Amazonian shamanism. In Indigenous Ayahuasca practices, Icaros are not merely background elements; they are dynamic tools that shape the course of the ceremony, illustrating the deep integration of music and spirituality in shamanic healing traditions.

The Differences between Indigenous and Western Practices

Indigenous Uses of Psychedelic Medicine

Exploring the differences between Indigenous and Western practices with Psychedelics is a deep and multifaceted topic. The contrast largely centers on the role and recognition of spirituality within the healing process (Luna and White, 2000).

In Indigenous cultures, such as those in the Amazon Basin using Ayahuasca, ceremonies occur in natural or community settings with spiritual interactions deeply embedded and seen as essential to the healing experience (Beyer, 2009). The spiritual beliefs integrated into their ceremonies dictate that health and sickness are not just about physical or mental states but are deeply influenced by spiritual balance (Graveline, 1998). Illness might be seen as a manifestation of spiritual disharmony or intrusion by harmful spirits, where spiritual interaction and intervention are considered crucial for achieving true healing (Dobkin de Rios and Rumrrill, 2008).

As already touched on, Icaros or sacred chants used within ceremonies are not merely songs; they are invocations that call upon spirits, ancestors, and other non-physical entities to participate in and guide the process of healing (Luna, 1984a). Indigenous shamans act as both spiritual guides and healers, believed to have powers and connections that are crucial for the ceremony's success.

There is a holistic view that considers physical, spiritual, mental, and communal health interconnected (Mabit, 2007; Wilson, 2008). The use of Psychedelics is not just about healing the individual but is seen as a way to maintain balance within the community and the natural world, where every element is interlinked. This is distinctly different from the Westernized use of Psychedelics, which often emphasizes psychological and therapeutic benefits without the same degree of spiritual or community engagement.

Westernized Uses of Psychedelic Medicine

In contrast, in Western settings, while the profound experiences induced by Psychedelics such as LSD, Ketamine, or MDMA are acknowledged, they are primarily framed within a psychological and medical model (Sessa, 2017). Psychedelics are administered in controlled settings like laboratories, clinics, or therapeutic sessions, often with medical oversight and under structured protocols to ensure safety and that effects can be measured scientifically (Carhart-Harris and Goodwin, 2017).

The use of these substances often focuses on their ability to provide deep personal insights, symptom relief, emotional release, or psychological transformation without the spiritual or communal aspects. These experiences are usually facilitated by therapists or researchers, where the goal is to support the individual's inner journey rather than to connect them with a spiritual world. In Western practices, the spiritual dimension, if recognized, is often considered a personal aspect of the experience rather than an intrinsic part of the psychedelic effect (Griffiths et al., 2008). The therapeutic framework is generally secular, and any spiritual experiences are viewed as subjective phenomena that contribute to the individual's personal growth.

Conclusion

Understanding these differences is crucial for respecting both approaches and for integrating Psychedelics into various cultural and medical frameworks thoughtfully and ethically. This dichotomy reflects broader differences in cultural understandings of mind, body, spirit, and healing, showing how cultural contexts shape the therapeutic use of psychedelic substances (Winkelman, 2010). Each approach offers unique insights and benefits, but they also highlight the need for cross-cultural sensitivity and respect in the global discourse on psychedelic therapy.

How the Western Renaissance with Psychedelic Medicines Affect Indigenous Communities

The "psychedelic renaissance" in Western cultures is significantly impacting Indigenous customs and communities. This movement, driven by a renewed interest in the therapeutic possibilities of Psychedelics such as psilocybin, MDMA, Ayahuasca, and LSD for mental health conditions like depression, PTSD, and anxiety, brings both potential benefits and significant challenges (Carhart-Harris and Goodwin, 2017).

Negative Consequences

Cultural Appropriation and Misrepresentation

The adoption of psychedelic substances in Western therapeutic and recreational settings often results in the dilution of the sacred rituals and culturally specific practices integral to their Indigenous use (Tupper, 2009). These profound traditions, refined over centuries, risk being reduced to mere commodities, stripped of their spiritual essence. Moreover, Western simplification and commercialization can lead to a homogenized and inaccurate portrayal of Indigenous practices, fostering widespread misunderstandings about the rich complexities and diversities of Indigenous cultures (Smith, 2012).

Economic Exploitation

The demand for psychedelic experiences has also sparked issues of biopiracy, where natural resources, including psychoactive plants, are exploited without just compensation or proper acknowledgment of the

Indigenous knowledge behind their discovery and use (Forte, 1997). Additionally, the rising trend of psychedelic tourism, especially to regions like the Amazon for Ayahuasca ceremonies, imposes significant pressures on local ecosystems and communities, potentially leading to the unsustainable harvesting of plants and disruption of Indigenous ways of life (Labate and Cavnar, 2014).

Legal and Ethical Issues

Disparities in regulation pose significant challenges as Western countries increasingly move toward the legalization or decriminalization of these substances, while Indigenous communities often remain bound by traditional laws that penalize their sacred practices (Miller, 2020). Additionally, ethical concerns arise regarding informed consent and benefit-sharing. Indigenous peoples frequently do not benefit from the commercialization of their traditional medicines and often have not provided genuine consent for the global use of their sacred practices (Shanon, 2010).

Impact on Indigenous Knowledge and Practices

Globalization threatens Indigenous sovereignty over their traditional knowledge and cultural heritage, risking the loss of ownership and control (Winkelman, 2010). The commodification of their sacred practices without appropriate cultural context jeopardizes the survival of these traditions, as central rituals and practices are commodified for external consumption (Gomez, 2020).

Potential Positive Impacts

On the brighter side, the psychedelic renaissance can enhance the recognition and respect for Indigenous knowledge, possibly encouraging initiatives to protect and preserve these traditions (Fotiou, 2016). It also opens avenues for cross-cultural dialogue about mental health, spirituality, and healing, fostering potentially more integrated approaches that honor both scientific and traditional knowledge (Mabit, 2007).

In conclusion, while the resurgence of interest in psychedelic medicines offers therapeutic prospects for Western societies, it is imperative to approach this renaissance with a deep awareness of its impacts on

Indigenous peoples. Ethical engagement, respect for cultural origins, and equitable benefit-sharing are crucial to mitigating negative effects and honoring the rich cultural legacies that have safeguarded these practices for generations.

Handling of Sacred Medicines

Handling and caring for sacred medicines—plant-based substances used in various spiritual and healing practices—requires a deep respect for their power and a clear understanding of their traditional uses (Beyer, 2009). These substances are considered sacred not only because of their psychoactive properties but also because they are seen as embodiments of spiritual entities or as gifts from the Earth that can teach, heal, and transform (Luna and White, 2000). How these medicines are approached and utilized can significantly influence their effectiveness and the safety of those who partake in their use.

Respect for Tradition

Many sacred medicines have been used for centuries within specific cultural rituals that involve prayers, songs, fasting, and other preparatory practices (Mabit, 2007). These traditions are designed to honor the spirit of medicine and prepare both the physical and spiritual bodies for the journey ahead. Ignoring these traditions can be disrespectful toward the cultures that have preserved these practices and potentially lead to dangerous outcomes for participants (Tupper, 2009).

Intention Setting

The intentions with which one approaches sacred medicines are believed to influence their effects (Shanon, 2010). Approaching these substances with humility, respect, and a genuine desire for healing or learning is considered crucial. Misuse or approaching these substances with intentions of power or greed can corrupt their effects and lead to harm (Harner, 1990).

Physical and Spiritual Safety

Proper handling ensures the physical and spiritual safety of those involved in the ceremonies. This includes knowing the correct dosages, understanding the physical and mental conditions that might contraindicate their use, and creating a safe, supportive environment for participants (Metzner, 1999). By understanding the profound responsibility associated with handling sacred medicines and actively working to prevent their misuse, individuals, and communities can help ensure that these practices continue to heal and enrich lives in the manner intended by their traditional custodians.

15

WHAT IS TRAUMA-INFORMED THERAPY USING A HARM-REDUCTION LENS?

Trauma-Informed Therapy

Trauma-informed therapy is an essential framework, particularly when supporting clients who are using Psychedelics for healing. This approach prioritizes creating a safe, supportive environment by recognizing the profound impact of trauma on the nervous system, fostering empowerment and choice, and minimizing the risk of re-traumatization (Levine, 2010). Such awareness is crucial, as many individuals seeking psychedelic therapy carry a history of trauma—experiences that often resurface during psychedelic journeys when clients are in an exceptionally vulnerable state (van der Kolk, 2014).

Why Trauma-Informed Therapy Is Essential in Psychedelic Healing

Psychedelic experiences can open up deep layers of the psyche, bringing to the surface past traumatic experiences that may not have been fully processed (Carhart-Harris et al., 2018b). This process can be immensely healing although potentially destabilizing if not handled with care. Trauma awareness is crucial for therapists to navigate these moments safely and effectively. According to Dr. Bessel van der Kolk in *The Body Keeps the Score* (2014), trauma affects both the body and mind, leading to physiological changes in the nervous system. During psychedelic

DOI: 10.4324/9781003595762-16

sessions, clients may relive traumatic memories, which can activate their fight-or-flight responses. Trauma-informed therapists help clients establish a sense of safety, enabling the therapeutic process to unfold without overwhelming them.

Guidelines and Techniques to Support Trauma-Informed Psychedelic Therapy

- **Identifying Possible Triggers**: In the preparation stages, it is important to discuss potential triggers with clients to anticipate and manage them during the session (Phelps, 2017). This foreknowledge allows therapists to intervene or support clients when distressing material arises.
- **Extended Duration of Sessions**: Psychedelic journeys can last significantly longer than traditional therapy sessions, often up to 6–8 hours or more. Therapists must prepare themselves for the increased vulnerability of clients during these extended periods and be present throughout to provide support and grounding (Gorman et al., 2021).
- **Connecting with Inner Resources**: Within preparation, inviting clients to connect with their inner sense of self, often referred to as "Self Energy" in Internal Family Systems (IFS) therapy (Schwartz, 2020b), can serve as a valuable resource during their journey. This sense of self can help them feel more empowered and less vulnerable when navigating challenging emotions and experiences.
- **Emphasizing Consent and Boundaries**: Discussing topics like consent, touch, safety cues, respecting boundaries, and confidentiality in advance is crucial. Establishing clear agreements fosters trust and ensures that clients feel safe throughout the experience. Pilecki et al. (2021) emphasize the importance of informed consent and maintaining a client-centered approach to support autonomy.
- **Ongoing Training**: Continued education in Trauma-informed approaches is necessary for therapists working in this field. Research in neuroscience and trauma treatment is rapidly evolving (Ogden et al., 2006), and staying informed ensures that therapists can provide the most up-to-date and effective support.

- **Cultural Sensitivity**: Therapists should be mindful of the client's cultural and spiritual background, as it significantly influences trauma healing (Harris and Fallot, 2001). Understanding the client's unique cultural perspective can help frame the psychedelic experience in a way that aligns with their beliefs and values.
- **Medical Considerations**: It is essential to assess medical or psychological conditions that could impact the safety of psychedelic use. Screening for mental health disorders, such as psychosis, which might contraindicate psychedelic therapy, is vital to prevent adverse outcomes (Johnson et al., 2008).

Harm Reduction Lens

Harm reduction is a pragmatic and compassionate approach to addressing substance use and other risky behaviors that focuses on minimizing negative consequences rather than promoting abstinence alone (Marlatt, 1996). When applied to psychedelic therapy, a harm reduction lens emphasizes safety, informed consent, integration support, and reducing potential risks while maximizing potential benefits (Gorman, 2018). This approach is particularly relevant in settings where psychedelic substances are used outside of a clinical context, such as underground therapy or personal exploration, where the risks can be more challenging to manage (Pilecki et al., 2021).

Harm reduction is based on the principle that providing clients with a nonjudgmental and supportive space is more effective than demanding strict adherence to abstinence or inducing feelings of shame (Marlatt, 1996). Therapists adopting a harm reduction approach work to build a trusting environment where clients feel safe to be open about their substance use. This method avoids pressuring clients into hiding their behaviors or terminating therapy due to fear of judgment.

In harm reduction, therapists maintain a non-coercive stance, helping clients assess the risks and benefits of their behaviors. By treating clients with dignity and respect, they are empowered to make informed decisions about their own lives. If complete abstinence is not a client's goal, the therapist may suggest alternatives, such as changing the route of administration, choosing a safer substance, adjusting surrounding behaviors, or reducing the frequency and intensity of use (Pilecki, B., et al., 2021).

Within this framework, therapists do not advocate either for or against psychedelic use (Pilecki, B., et al. 2021). Instead, they focus on the client's overall well-being and desired outcomes, facilitating a process where clients can explore what actions will support the life they envision. Often, this involves helping the client clarify their motivations for seeking psychedelic experiences. The therapist might then propose alternative options for achieving the client's goals, such as alternative methods of achieving altered states of consciousness like focussing meditation, breathwork, traditional psychotherapy/Art Therapy, participation in FDA (Food and Drug Administration)-approved psychedelic trials, or other legal means. The key is presenting these options in an unbiased manner, allowing clients to make informed decisions that align with their values and circumstances.

When applying a harm reduction lens in psychedelic therapy, there is a focus on developing internal skills and tools through the integration process after an experience, ensuring that chronic use of the medicine does not become the focus of healing (Johnson et al., 2008). Many who experience psychedelic medicines express the notion of a window into the psyche opening that allows for more expansive healing to take place afterward. Pilecki, B., et al. (2021) highlight that this approach also involves ethical considerations around client autonomy, informed consent, and the non-judgmental support of clients' choices, whether they involve continued use of Psychedelics or not.

Although Psychedelics are generally not considered addictive, seeking out heightened experiences can become problematic (Garcia-Romeu et al., 2014). This is why harm reduction is so important in this work. It counters the current trend toward capitalization and monetization of psychedelic enterprise by shifting the focus from ongoing engagement with the medicine to the work of integration and healing that comes from within after having had a psychedelic experience. Pilecki, B., et al. (2021) emphasize the role of therapists in providing integration services that address the potential psychological and existential challenges clients may encounter post-experience. They advocate for a nuanced approach that acknowledges the potential risks of Psychedelics, such as psychological distress or the exacerbation of mental health symptoms, and the importance of providing clients with supportive spaces to process their experiences.

In practice, therapists using a harm reduction lens might engage in discussions with clients about safe use practices, help them prepare for the experience, and offer post-experience integration support to foster long-term benefits while minimizing harm. Pilecki et al. (2021) also address the legal complexities therapists face when working in jurisdictions where psychedelic use remains illegal, advocating for careful navigation of these ethical and legal boundaries to support clients effectively.

16
THREE-STAGE MODEL OF TRAUMA THERAPY

Judith Herman first introduced the three-phase model of trauma therapy in her groundbreaking book *Trauma and Recovery* (1992). Rooted in a person-centered, feminist approach, this model honors the lived experiences of trauma survivors. Central to the framework is the creation of safety and stabilization, providing clients with a secure foundation to explore, process, and ultimately transcend the effects of trauma and symptoms of Post-Traumatic Stress Disorder (PTSD). Over time, this model has been adopted and expanded by leading trauma experts, including Bessel van der Kolk (2014), Cathy Malchiodi (2015), Peter Levine (Levine and Frederick, 1997), and Christine Courtois (2004). Due to its widespread acceptance and application, it is often referred to as the *Consensus Model* (McEvoy and Ziegler, 2006).

Stage One: Safety and Stabilization

This stage involves working toward internal and external safety for the client. It begins by building a therapeutic alliance with the therapist so the client feels safe to move forward. Some areas that may be focused on in this stage are understanding the impacts of trauma and violence, personal self-care, addressing problems with alcohol or drugs, depression, eating behaviors, self-harming behaviors, physical health, panic attacks,

DOI: 10.4324/9781003595762-17

dissociation, and especially developing and strengthening skills to increase one's capacity to manage and minimize unhealthy responses to painful and unwanted emotions and flashbacks (Herman, 1992). Through learning these skills, the client becomes more secure in the internal power they hold to heal.

Tapping into and developing one's inner strengths and any other potentially available resources for healing is very important in the healing journey. Relationships in the client's life may be explored to ensure that they are safe and supported (McEvoy and Ziegler, 2006). Treatment goals are also discussed with a focus on various approaches that may be used to assist in reaching these.

During this stage of therapy, discussing a client's memories should not be the focus of therapy but a means to achieving safety, stability, and a greater ability to take care of oneself. Especially if memories of abusive experiences are repressed, it is important in the first stage of recovery and treatment that they are not discussed or processed (Herman, 1992). However, everything is not always perfectly ordered and sequential. It may be necessary to discuss parts of disturbing memories when they are disrupting one's life so the client is able to manage them.

There is a delicate balance within the therapeutic relationship that needs to be observed; by going too fast when working with trauma survivors, the therapist may be put in the role of the perpetrator if they present as intrusive or investigative in their manner and approach. However, by going too slow, the therapist may put themselves in the role of the passive bystander who sees but says nothing (McEvoy and Ziegler, 2006). Both of these approaches can recapitulate the trauma within the therapeutic setting.

Because the tasks of the first stage of recovery are arduous and demanding, patients and therapists alike frequently try to bypass them. It is often tempting to overlook the requirement of safety and to rush headlong into the later stages of therapeutic work. Though the single most common therapeutic error is the avoidance of the traumatic material, probably the second most common error is premature or precipitate engagement in exploratory work, without sufficient attention to the tasks of establishing safety and securing a therapeutic alliance (Herman, 1992).

Once these 'stage-one' goals of building capacity for personal safety, genuine self-care, and healthy emotion regulation have become standard operating procedures, great progress and many new choices become possible.

Stage Two: Remembrance and Mourning

When safety and stabilization have been achieved, trauma therapy moves into the second stage, which addresses the deeper impact of trauma by processing and integrating the traumatic experiences. It becomes a time of grief and mourning (Herman, 1992) as clients begin to deconstruct negative beliefs that have formed within them as a result of the trauma (Roth et al., 1997), and work to develop positive schemas or beliefs (McCann and Pearlman, 1990).

As this stage continues, clients work to alleviate their post-traumatic symptoms by actively intervening when they arise (Briere, 2002). By reviewing and discussing memories that have happened in their past, they begin to lessen the emotional intensity that is brought on by these memories. This is best done once the client feels safe, resourced, and secure. Through this experience, the client also begins to revise the meanings of their life and identity. They reconstruct the effect their traumas have had on them. They are able to face their experiences, which could also include mourning for experiences they did not have but wished for, like secure attachment or love (van der Kolk, 2014). It is in the therapeutic relationship that this can be explored as the client fosters the ability and inner resources to accept their life and feel the strength within to deal with the pains of their past.

However, sometimes after the first stage of therapy has laid out a foundation of safety and stability, a client may discover that thinking and talking about painful memories is not necessary to achieve their goals. If they find that the memories are no longer disrupting their life, the therapist needs to honor what the client feels they need and be sensitive to their reasons for not wanting to explore the trauma.

For those who choose to direct their attention to the disturbing memories that are still disrupting their lives, several memory-processing methods can be used, including Eye Movement Desensitization and Reprocessing (EMDR) (van der Kolk, 2014, p. 183). We will further explore this approach in part two of this book, outlining the theoretical aspects of using EMDR in combination with Art Therapy to support this second stage of trauma therapy within psychedelic-assisted therapy.

Stage Three: Acceptance and Reintegration into Ordinary Life

The third stage of recovery focuses on reconnecting with people, meaningful activities, and other aspects of life. "This is a time for reconnection with others and with ordinary life" (Herman, 1992, p. 155). During this stage, the therapist becomes a sounding board as the survivor practices new learnings and behaviors and builds new experiences (McEvoy and Ziegler, 2006). By this point, they will have developed their internal strengths and resources. When the therapy moves into this stage where the therapist listens and holds the space rather than actively working to help stabilize the client, the client feels more empowered, which is one of the main focuses in this feminist-based model of trauma therapy (Herman, 1992).

Common to All Stages

As mentioned, these stages are not always concurrent. The therapeutic process may vacillate from one stage to another and then back again to an earlier stage. The healing journey needs to be adaptive to the needs of the client. Throughout all stages of treatment, it is often necessary to address psychological themes related to one's history of unwanted or abusive experiences. Some of these are core issues that will determine the nature and structure of treatment. They include:

1. Powerlessness
2. Shame and guilt
3. Distrust
4. Re-enacting abusive patterns in current relationships (Herman, 1992)

When these themes and dynamics are obstacles to safety, self-care, and regulating one's emotions and behavior, they must be addressed in the first stage of treatment before the client is able to move into the following stages (McEvoy and Ziegler, 2006).

With the help of therapy, the client is encouraged to recognize habitual behavior patterns they possess and then shift them so they no longer engage in self-defeating and self-destructive behaviors that are outside of their conscious awareness. By increasing awareness of these themes and dynamics, the client develops a clearer understanding of them and becomes able to take responsibility for them when they arise, which in turn gives them the capacity to choose new, healthier responses and actions (Herman, 1992).

17

SUICIDE AND PSYCHEDELICS

The relationship between psychedelic use and suicide is intricate, influenced by factors such as an individual's mental health history, the context in which Psychedelics are used, and the intentions behind their use. Research on this topic is expanding, revealing both potential risks and therapeutic benefits (Carhart-Harris and Goodwin, 2017).

Connection between Psychedelics and Suicide Risk

Potential Decrease in Suicide Risk

- **Therapeutic Benefits**: Emerging research suggests that Psychedelics, when administered in controlled, therapeutic settings, can significantly reduce symptoms of depression, anxiety, and PTSD—common risk factors for suicide. For instance, studies involving psilocybin and LSD indicate that, when combined with therapy, these substances can provide deep emotional relief, leading to an improved mood and reduced suicidal thoughts (Griffiths et al., 2016; Ross et al., 2016).
- **Sense of Connectedness:** Psychedelic experiences often foster feelings of interconnectedness and reduce isolation, a key factor in suicidal ideation. This heightened sense of belonging and purpose can contribute to a lower risk of suicide (Watts et al., 2017).

DOI: 10.4324/9781003595762-18

In a study by Carhart-Harris et al. (2018c), participants reported enhanced feelings of connection to others and the world, which contributed to positive shifts in their mental health.

Potential Increase in Suicide Risk

- **Challenging Experiences:** While many find psychedelic experiences enlightening, others can encounter distressing effects, such as anxiety, fear, and confusion. These challenging experiences can exacerbate underlying mental health conditions, particularly if not properly managed in a supportive setting (Johnson et al., 2008).
- **Unregulated Use:** When Psychedelics are used outside of a therapeutic context, particularly by individuals with unresolved trauma or co-occurring mental health disorders, outcomes can be unpredictable and potentially harmful (Garcia-Romeu et al., 2014). Such unregulated use may result in increased distress or destabilization.
- **"Magic Bullet" Beliefs**: Some individuals view Psychedelics as a last resort or a "magic bullet" to solve their mental health issues. While psychedelic substances can open a window to deep healing, it is the integration process that facilitates lasting change. The expectation that Psychedelics will provide a cure can lead to profound disappointment if the experience does not meet these hopes, potentially resulting in increased suicide risk. Pilecki et al. (2021) highlight the importance of integration to help individuals process their experiences and avoid feelings of hopelessness that might arise if immediate change is not apparent.

Prevalence of Suicide among Psychedelic Users

Due to the legal status of Psychedelics in many regions, there is limited structured research on the prevalence of suicide among those using these substances. However, anecdotal evidence and preliminary studies suggest that therapeutic use of Psychedelics, when properly managed, is generally associated with a decrease in suicidal ideation (Griffiths et al., 2016). This contrasts with potential risks that might be linked to recreational or unsupervised use.

Preventing Suicide in Psychedelic Therapy

Screening and Preparation

Conduct comprehensive psychological assessments to evaluate suicide risk and other mental health concerns before beginning psychedelic therapy (Johnson et al., 2008).

Prepare participants for the experience by setting realistic expectations and discussing potential emotional challenges that may arise (Phelps, 2017).

1. **Professional Supervision:**
   - Ensure psychedelic sessions are conducted by trained professionals who can offer immediate support and intervene during moments of distress (Mithoefer et al., 2016).
   - Utilize integration therapists to help clients process their experiences post-session constructively.
2. **Follow-Up Care:**
   - Provide thorough aftercare, including regular check-ins and support group meetings, to monitor participants' mental health.
   - Develop a safety plan with warning signs, coping strategies, and emergency contact information.
3. **Creating a Supportive Setting:**
   - Conduct sessions in a secure, comfortable environment to reduce anxiety and promote a positive experience (Carhart-Harris et al., 2018b).
   - Encourage a support network of family or friends who understand the participant's therapeutic goals.
4. **Integration Work:**
   - Offer ongoing integration sessions to help participants make sense of their psychedelic experiences and apply insights to everyday life (Watts et al., 2017). Integration is a crucial step for fostering meaningful change and mitigating risks.

Conclusion

While the use of Psychedelics carries the potential for both positive and negative impacts on suicide risk, careful management, and professional oversight are key. Therapeutic use of these substances, when conducted according to best practices, shows promise in reducing symptoms of depression, anxiety, and suicidal ideation. Ongoing research and clinical trials will help refine these approaches, maximizing benefits while minimizing risks.

PART II
THE PROCESS

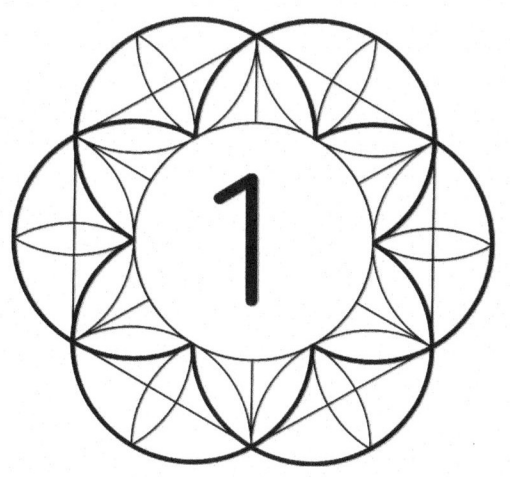

MODULE 1
PREPARING FOR A PSYCHEDELIC EXPERIENCE

Just as important as the integration process after a psychedelic experience is the preparation process. Having a sense of what you may encounter and strategies for navigating difficult moments can significantly influence the quality and depth of your journey. Using Psychedelics for healing is a profound practice that deserves careful consideration. Many Psychedelics are derived from ancient Indigenous medicines, carrying cultural and spiritual significance that must be honored and respected. Even when administered by a medical professional in a clinical setting, understanding what may arise and how to approach it is imperative.

This chapter provides practical tools to support your experience, including thoughtful guidelines, easy-to-follow art directives, and meditative practices. No formal art training is required to engage with the art directives in this book—they are designed to help you connect with internal sensations and access unconscious insights. The focus is on the process of creation, not the final product.

Consider the following elements to support your journey:

1. Setting an Intention
2. Practicing Meditation

DOI: 10.4324/9781003595762-20

3. Maintaining a Clean Diet Beforehand
4. Using Supportive Tools During Your Journey
5. Creating a Plan for Post-Journey Integration

Creating Set and Setting

Set and setting refer to the psychological and environmental factors that influence the psychedelic experience. Ensuring that the set (the mindset, intentions, beliefs, and emotional state of the individual) and the setting (the physical environment in which the journey is taking place, social context, and interpersonal dynamics) feel comfortable and safe is essential for promoting a positive and transformative psychedelic experience (Leary, 1964). Knowing these factors is an effective way to feel a bit of agency and control before entering into such a vulnerable state.

Preparing with Art Therapy

Throughout this book, you are invited to begin using the creative process as a way to connect to your own feelings, emotions, and intentions before, during, and after your experience. As referenced over and again, art and seeing the world through a creative and exploratory lens has always been a part of psychedelic journeys. Art Therapy can be a valuable tool for preparing for a psychedelic journey by helping to access, explore, and express intentions, fears, and hopes about the experience about to be undertaken. The creations you make in your preparation can be guides to support you throughout the process of psychedelic therapy, as a reminder of the connection you have with Self, inner strength, and the resilience you hold within.

Preparing with Meditation

Do you already have a meditation practice? Regulating our emotions through focused attention and conscious breathing can be invaluable tools as we prepare for a psychedelic journey. During such experiences, it's common to feel overwhelmed, making it essential to have strategies for self-regulation. Regularly engaging in meditative or mindfulness practices beforehand helps establish a grounding presence within the psyche—one that you can reliably draw upon when needed.

In this module, you'll find some exercises to try. If you already have a favorite practice, I invite you to begin using it consistently at least a couple of weeks before your journey. Regular meditation helps to rewire neural pathways in the brain, enhancing our ability to focus and self-regulate. The more we practice, the quicker we can calm the mind and support the body and nervous system with greater ease.

However, not everyone finds it easy to access bodily awareness. For some, focusing on subtle internal sensations can feel dysregulating and deeply uncomfortable. This is especially true for individuals who have experienced trauma, where tuning into the body may feel unsafe. In such cases, dissociation can become a coping mechanism for navigating the world. It's crucial to be mindful of this—we don't want meditation to trigger anxiety or distress.

For clients who experience difficulty, I often begin with a gentle approach by inviting awareness to a specific body part, such as the left big toe. Simply noticing the sensations in this area and focusing attention on it can foster a sense of grounding, creating space for a mindful practice that feels safe and approachable. Remember, everyone is different, so take the time to honor how you feel and what you need. This act of self-awareness is a valuable practice in itself—one that we will continue to nurture throughout the preparation stage.

There are many different types of meditation, so find one that feels accessible and works for you. It's not about meditating for an hour every day—if you can, that's wonderful, but it's not required. Even starting with just 3–11 minutes at a consistent time each day can help you establish a regular practice. What's most important in the beginning is setting realistic goals that feel achievable. Start small if that feels right, and gradually build from there, honoring your own pace and process.

Within this book, I offer many guided meditations for you to explore. To begin, I invite you to:

- **Become aware of your breath,** noticing the gentle rise and fall as it moves through your body.
- **Feel the surface beneath you,** observing where your body makes contact with it. This practice enhances both tactile awareness and proprioception, helping to ground you in the present moment.
- **Gently expand and soften your breath,** allowing for deeper relaxation with every exhale.

- **Notice the subtle pause** at the top of each inhale and the bottom of each exhale. What does it feel like to rest briefly in these quiet spaces?
- **Count the seconds** of your inhales and exhales if it feels helpful, supporting a steady, even rhythm in your breathing.
- **Begin with a light body scan,** gently noticing any areas of tension or discomfort. Imagine your breath as a liquid light flowing into these spaces—clearing and expanding with each inhale, releasing and dissolving tension with each exhale. Feel the surface beneath you, and allow the earth to absorb anything that no longer serves you, creating space within for ease and clarity.

Continue your meditation practice in the weeks leading up to your psychedelic journey to help clear the mind and cultivate tools that will support you during the experience. As you meditate, gently begin to focus on an intention you'd like to carry into your journey. What are you hoping to receive from this experience? What are you seeking to heal, discover, or uncover? As you create space within your psyche and unconscious, notice any feelings or thoughts that rise to the surface. Acknowledge them with curiosity and compassion, then gently return your awareness to the breath.

Art Directive: Preparing with Intention

Before embarking on a psychedelic journey, it's helpful to reflect on the intention you'd like to set. This intention could focus on an area of your life you're working on, insights that support personal growth, healing past traumas, deepening your connection to universal energy, enhancing spiritual development, or expanding consciousness.

This directive is intentionally open-ended, allowing you to define your personal intention. Once you've identified it, you're invited to create an image that represents this intention. Approach the process spontaneously, staying open to whatever arises—whether subtle bodily sensations, memories, emotions, or unexpected associations (Carpendale, 2009).

Materials Needed
- Paper in any size or shape of your choosing
- Ample materials to choose from including:
  - Markers
  - Pencil crayons
  - Watercolor paints
  - Acrylic paints
  - Crayons
  - Oils pastels
  - Chalk pastels

After a brief centering in the body or meditation, find a spot that feels safe and comfortable. Set the setting with candles, incense, soft music or whatever feels supportive for your environment. It's important to be in a space that you will not be disturbed.

Begin moving materials on the page, working in a way that taps into the intuitive side of you as you choose which materials want to be used. As you continue to move materials bring your intention for your journey to mind and create that. Staying connected to the breath and feeling the feet on the ground. Notice what emerges and wants to be spoken of through the art. Trust your process and that you are being supported to allow for the most poignant information that will support your journey.

After finishing your creation, take some time to reflect by placing your image at a distance from you and noticing the feelings that come up within the body. Begin a dialogue with your art taking notes in your journal in whatever way feels important.

Automatic Writing/Journaling

Incorporating journaling after meditation or art making can be a powerful way to explore insights that surface. Allow your pen to move freely across the page without judgment or attachment to the words being written. This technique, known as **automatic writing**, helps access the unconscious mind, bringing hidden thoughts, feelings, and wisdom to light (Braud, 2003). Making this a regular practice can be especially valuable in preparing for a psychedelic journey, as it fosters deeper self-reflection and connection with your inner world.

Consider visualizing different parts of yourself, much like how you experience various moods or emotions. Invite these parts to express themselves through your writing. This approach aligns with the **Internal Family Systems (IFS) model**, which encourages exploration of inner voices or "parts" to promote self-awareness and healing (Schwartz, 2020b).

If you hold a belief in something greater than yourself—whether it's angels, guides, your higher self, source energy, nature, or a deity—connecting with this energy can offer additional support. For example, imagine reaching out to your higher self or Soul. Use one color of pen to write a question you'd like guidance on, then take a deep, centering breath. With another color, begin automatic writing as if channeling wisdom from this higher source. This process can feel both supportive and empowering. To deepen the practice, consider using your non-dominant hand to respond, as this can help access different layers of consciousness (Capacchione,1988).

Throughout this practice, stay attuned to your breath, bodily sensations, and any emotions that arise. This mindful awareness helps you connect with different aspects of yourself, offering clarity as you reflect on your intentions for the psychedelic journey. Keep an open mind to whatever intuitive messages emerge, and gently explore what you hope to gain, heal, or discover along the way.

Foods to Avoid before Your Psychedelic Experience

Certain foods are recommended to avoid before a psychedelic healing journey, as they may interfere with the experience or cause physical discomfort (Fadiman, 2011). The dietary restrictions vary depending on the type of psychedelic, with some substances requiring stricter preparation than others. However, it is generally a good practice to avoid the following items:

1. **Monoamine Oxidase Inhibitors (MAOIs)**: Psilocybin is metabolized into psilocin, with minor involvement of monoamine oxidase (MAO). While psilocybin alone doesn't require dietary restrictions, combining it with MAOIs (pharmaceutical or natural) can increase the intensity and duration of psilocybin's

effects by slowing down its breakdown in the body. Additionally, if MAOIs are involved, consuming tyramine-rich foods—such as aged cheeses, fermented products (sauerkraut, soy sauce), cured meats, bananas, and avocados—can cause dangerous spikes in blood pressure (Tylš et al., 2014). If you are not taking an MAOI, these food restrictions do not apply.

2. **Heavy or Processed Foods:** Eating heavy or processed foods can lead to digestive discomfort and a sluggish feeling, potentially detracting from the clarity of the psychedelic experience (Fadiman, 2011). It is advisable to consume light, fresh, and easily digestible foods. A balanced meal consisting of fruits, vegetables, whole grains, and lean proteins is typically recommended.

3. **Caffeine and Stimulants:** Foods and beverages containing caffeine (such as coffee, tea, energy drinks, and chocolate) are stimulants that may increase anxiety and restlessness or intensify the effects of Psychedelics, such as psilocybin (Johnson et al., 2008). It is recommended to avoid or limit caffeine consumption prior to the journey to maintain a calmer state of mind.

4. **Spicy or Heavy Seasoning:** Spicy or heavily seasoned foods can sometimes lead to gastrointestinal discomfort, which may be amplified during the psychedelic experience (Fadiman, 2011). Opting for milder flavors, especially for those prone to digestive sensitivity, can help avoid unnecessary distractions or discomfort.

5. **Excessive Sugar:** High sugar intake can cause energy fluctuations, mood swings, and potential crashes, which can affect the stability of the experience. Minimizing sugary foods and beverages before the journey helps maintain steady energy levels (Tupper, 2008).

6. **Large or Heavy Meals:** Consuming a large or heavy meal before a psychedelic experience may lead to discomfort, digestive issues, or a feeling of sluggishness. It is generally recommended to eat a light and nutritious meal a few hours before the journey to ensure sufficient energy without causing digestive distress (Mithoefer et al., 2016).

It is important to remember that individual sensitivities and dietary preferences vary. Listening to your body and making choices that support your well-being is essential. Since different substances interact with foods in various ways, exercising caution is advisable. Prioritizing a nourishing and balanced diet leading up to the experience can promote both physical and mental clarity. If you have specific dietary concerns or restrictions, consulting a healthcare professional or nutritionist for personalized guidance is recommended.

Drugs, Alcohol, and Supplements to Avoid

1. **Alcohol**: Avoiding alcohol before a psychedelic experience is crucial, as it can impair judgment and interact unpredictably with the effects of psychedelic substances (Mithoefer et al., 2016). Alcohol's depressant effects can conflict with the typically mind-expanding nature of Psychedelics, leading to confusion and potential emotional dysregulation.

2. **Recreational Drugs:** It is important to refrain from using recreational drugs, such as cannabis, cocaine, amphetamines, or other substances that may alter perception or cognition. Mixing Psychedelics with these substances can result in unpredictable and potentially dangerous interactions (Fadiman, 2011). While some practitioners use cannabis psychoactively in certain settings, taking a break from regular usage before a psychedelic ceremony is advisable to allow for a "clean slate" and maximize the intended effects of the experience.

3. **Prescription Medications:** Certain prescription medications can interact negatively with Psychedelics. Consulting a healthcare professional, particularly one knowledgeable about psychedelic substances, is key to ensuring safety. They can provide guidance on whether it is safe to continue or adjust any current medication regimen before the experience (Johnson et al., 2008).

4. **SSRI Antidepressants:** Selective serotonin reuptake inhibitors (SSRIs) and similar antidepressants can either diminish the effects of Psychedelics or cause adverse reactions due to their impact on serotonin levels in the brain (Carhart-Harris and Goodwin, 2017). If you are on SSRIs, it is important to discuss

with your prescribing doctor the possibility of gradually discontinuing the medication before considering a psychedelic journey, ensuring a safe transition and minimizing potential risks.

5. **MAOI Medications:** Monoamine oxidase inhibitors (MAOIs) are a class of antidepressants that can have serious interactions with certain Psychedelics, particularly those containing DMT, such as Ayahuasca (Tylš et al., 2014). MAOIs can significantly increase the potency and duration of Psychedelics, potentially leading to severe complications. It is critical to avoid MAOIs for an appropriate period before a psychedelic journey and to follow the guidance of a healthcare professional.

6. **Stimulants:** Substances like caffeine, amphetamines, and other stimulants can increase anxiety, heart rate, and blood pressure. Combining these with Psychedelics can intensify stimulation, leading to restlessness or discomfort (Johnson et al., 2008). To maintain a calm and balanced state, it is best to avoid these substances before the experience.

7. **Certain Herbal Supplements:** Herbal supplements, such as St. John's Wort and valerian root, can interact with Psychedelics and potentially alter mood or perception. It is crucial to research potential interactions and consult a healthcare professional if you have concerns about specific supplements you are taking (Tupper, 2008).

Because individual sensitivities and drug interactions vary, consulting with a healthcare professional experienced with Psychedelics is recommended. If discussing with your doctor is not an option, a pharmacist can often assist in identifying contraindications. Given the varied interactions between substances, exercising caution is always the best approach to ensure a safe and beneficial psychedelic experience.

How to Avoid a "Bad Trip"

Adverse Psychedelic Experiences

An adverse psychedelic experience, commonly known as a "bad" or "challenging" trip, can result from various factors, including an individual's mindset, the setting, the substance used, inadequate physical preparation (such as diet and refraining from other substances), and not cleansing the body of contraindicating medications (Johnson et al., 2008). Understanding and addressing these factors can significantly minimize the likelihood of a challenging experience.

Careful Planning of Set and Setting

- **Mindset Preparation:** Before the experience, engage in practices that promote a positive mindset, such as meditation, self-reflection, or guided visualization. Address any current mental health issues with a therapist to prepare emotionally (Carhart-Harris et al., 2018b).
- **Choose the Right Environment:** Ensure the environment is safe, comfortable, and familiar. Being in a quiet, controlled space where external stressors are minimized can help create a more positive experience (Leary et al., 1964).

Appropriate Dosage and Substance Knowledge

- **Consult an Expert:** Work with a knowledgeable guide or therapist who can advise on the correct dosage and ensure the substance is safe and pure. This professional insight is crucial for ensuring a safe experience (Mithoefer et al., 2016).
- **Start Low:** Begin with a lower dose, especially if it is your first experience or you are trying a new substance. This cautious approach allows you to gauge how your body and mind respond.

Professional or Experienced Guidance

- **Supervised Experiences:** Whenever possible, have the experience under the supervision of a trained therapist or experienced guide. They can provide emotional support and guidance, helping to navigate difficult thoughts or emotions that may arise during the journey (Griffiths et al., 2016).

Physical Well-Being

- **Physical Readiness:** Ensure that you are physically well, meaning you are well-rested, hydrated, and have eaten nourishing foods. Refraining from drugs, alcohol, sex, and certain foods (depending on the substance) can help clear the mind, body, and psyche to withstand the intensity of a psychedelic experience (Fadiman, 2011).

- **Energetic Diet:** Some Indigenous teachings recommend an "energetic diet" before ceremonies, which involves abstaining from sexual gratification, gossip, and negative thoughts to maintain a clear and focused mindset (Tupper, 2008).

Education and Intentions

- **Educate Yourself:** Learning about what to expect during a psychedelic experience can reduce fear and anxiety. Understanding the range of possible sensations and thoughts prepares you mentally for what may come (Grof, 1980b).
- **Set Intentions:** Clearly define your intentions for the experience. Having a purpose can serve as a touchstone if the journey becomes challenging.

Negative Spirits (Bruja Energy)

- **Spiritual Protection:** According to Indigenous teachings, negative energies (brujas) can infiltrate a ceremony if it is not properly contained in a sacred manner (Metzner, 1999). It is vital to ensure that any shaman or facilitator you work with is adequately trained to create a protective sacred space for participants.

Integration Preparation

- **Plan for Integration:** Knowing in advance that you will have support for processing and understanding your experience, whether through a therapist or support group, can provide reassurance and help with post-experience integration (Phelps, 2017).

Emergency Plan

- **Prepare for Intensity:** Have a plan in place to manage intense experiences, which might include a calming music playlist, a list of contacts for immediate support, or a comfortable retreat space.

Proper preparation can significantly reduce the risk of a "bad trip" by creating a feeling of safety and support. While it's impossible to guarantee that a challenging experience won't occur, these preparations can help mitigate adverse reactions and support a more constructive outcome.

Supporting a "Bad Trip"

When navigating a challenging or "bad" trip, it is crucial to approach the situation with compassion, mindfulness, and the intention of creating a safe and grounded environment. Here are some gentle, heart-centered steps to help you through this experience.

Stay Calm and Present

- **Remain Calm:** Your calm presence can act as a stabilizing force amid emotional turbulence. Imagining yourself as a serene anchor in the storm of emotions can create an inner ripple of peace (Grof, 1980a). By maintaining a sense of calm, you can foster a space where healing and processing can occur.

Ensure Physical Safety

- **Create a Safe Space:** Find a comfortable place where you feel protected. Remove any potentially hazardous objects and cocoon yourself in a comforting environment. Knowing that you are physically safe allows you to relax more deeply into the experience (Johnson et al., 2008).

Use Grounding Techniques

- **Connect with the Present Moment:** Focus on your breath, the sensation of the ground beneath you, or hold a comforting object that helps anchor you in the present. Grounding techniques, such as mindful breathing, can reduce feelings of disorientation and panic, helping you to remain centered during intense moments (Kabat-Zinn, 1990).

Offer Supportive Self-Talk

- **Speak Kindly to Yourself:** Acknowledge the intensity of your experience while reminding yourself that it is temporary and that you are safe. Supportive self-talk can soothe your mind, reduce fear, and help you feel more connected to your inner strength (Polster and Polster, 1973).

Adjust the Environment

- **Create a Calming Atmosphere:** Adjust your surroundings to reduce sensory overload. Dim the lights, wrap yourself in a blanket, or move to a quieter space if needed. A soothing environment can help you feel more secure (Mithoefer et al., 2016).
- **Change Your Position:** If you are lying down, consider sitting up to alter your physical state, which may alleviate the intensity of your feelings.
- **Remove or Adjust Sensory Input:** If you have a blindfold on, removing it to let light in can help ease an intense experience. Similarly, changing evocative music to something more calming can significantly affect the journey's direction, as music profoundly influences emotional states during psychedelic experiences (Kaelen et al., 2018).

Face Your Fears

- **Engage with Frightening Imagery:** When encountering intense visionary experiences, such as frightening beings or objects, consider facing the imagery directly and asking if it is your teacher. This approach, discussed in Joseph Tafur's *Fellowship of the River* (Tafur, 2017), can help transform potentially distressing experiences into opportunities for insight and healing. If the imagery is not a teacher, it will often vanish; if it is, it may morph into something offering valuable guidance.

Bring Back Your Resource Image

- In Module 3, you are invited to connect with an inner resource and create a representation of this. This resource image can serve as an anchor, reminding you of your resilience and capabilities. Visualizing this image can help restore a sense of stability and empowerment (Levine, 2010; Schaverien, 1992).

Navigating a challenging psychedelic experience can be daunting, but with compassion, mindfulness, and proper support, it can transform into a profound opportunity for growth. Remember to stay grounded, ensure your safety, and seek guidance when needed. These challenging experiences, although difficult, can be turned into powerful catalysts for self-discovery and transformation.

What Is Serotonin Syndrome?

Serotonin Syndrome, also known as serotonin toxicity or serotonin sickness, is a potentially life-threatening condition that arises from an excessive accumulation of serotonin in the body. This can occur when medications or substances that affect serotonin levels are taken together (Boyer and Shannon, 2005). Since many Psychedelics also influence serotonin receptors, the risk of serotonin syndrome is especially relevant when combined with certain pharmaceutical medications.

Causes of Serotonin Syndrome

- **Combination of Serotonergic Medications:** The use of antidepressants like SSRIs, SNRIs (Serotonin-Norepinephrine Reuptake Inhibitors), certain pain medications, and anti-migraine drugs alongside other serotonin-elevating substances increases the risk (Volpi-Abadie et al., 2013).
- **Interaction with Psychedelics:** Classic Psychedelics, including LSD, psilocybin, and DMT, act on serotonin receptors, particularly the 5-HT2A receptor. When these are taken with other serotonergic drugs, they can exacerbate the risk of serotonin syndrome (Nichols, 2016).

Symptoms of Serotonin Syndrome

Symptoms can appear within hours of drug interaction and vary from mild to severe. They include:

- **Cognitive Effects:** Confusion, agitation, hypomania, hallucinations, and headaches.
- **Autonomic Effects:** Fever, sweating, shivering, accelerated heart rate, and high blood pressure (Boyer and Shannon, 2005).

- **Somatic Effects:** Dilated pupils, muscle rigidity, twitching, coordination problems, and muscle spasms.
- **Gastrointestinal Symptoms:** Nausea, vomiting, and diarrhea.
- **Catatonic States:** Severe cases can lead to catatonic states, particularly when combining certain pharmaceutical medications (like those used for depression and psychosis) with Psychedelics such as ibogaine (Wilcox et al., 2014).

Severe serotonin syndrome can be life-threatening, potentially causing seizures, irregular heartbeat, or extreme hyperthermia, and may require emergency medical intervention.

Prevention and Management

Preventing serotonin syndrome involves careful management of medications and substances affecting serotonin levels:

- **Medication Review:** Before starting any new medication or psychedelic substance, reviewing current medications with a healthcare provider is crucial. This includes prescription drugs, over-the-counter medications, dietary supplements, and illicit substances (Boyer and Shannon, 2005).
- **Avoid Certain Combinations**: Refrain from mixing SSRIs, SNRIs, MAOIs, or TCAs with Psychedelics without medical advice. These medications impact serotonin levels, and their interaction with Psychedelics can be unpredictable and dangerous (Nichols, 2016).
- **Monitor Dosages and Responses:** If combining substances under medical guidance, it is important to begin with low dosages and monitor the body's response to avoid excessive serotonin accumulation.
- **Education and Awareness:** Being informed about the symptoms of serotonin syndrome enables early detection and intervention, reducing the risk of severe outcomes (Volpi-Abadie et al., 2013).

Treatment for Serotonin Syndrome

Treatment strategies typically involve:

- **Stopping Serotonergic Drugs:** Immediately discontinuing any drugs suspected of contributing to the syndrome.
- **Supportive Care:** This includes managing agitation with sedatives, controlling autonomic instability (such as blood pressure and temperature), and ensuring adequate hydration.
- **Medications:** In severe cases, serotonin antagonists like cyproheptadine may be used to block serotonin production (Boyer and Shannon, 2005).
- **Hospitalization:** For severe cases involving extreme hyperthermia or cardiac disturbances, hospitalization may be necessary for intensive monitoring and intervention.

Serotonin syndrome is a serious condition that requires awareness, cautious management of serotonergic substances, and prompt medical attention when symptoms arise.

Different Psychoactive Drugs, Their Origins, Contraindications, and Precautions

Organic Psychedelic Drugs

1. **Psilocybin:**
   - **Origin:** Found in certain species of mushrooms, known as "magic mushrooms" or "shrooms." They grow primarily in Central and South America, North America, Europe, Asia, and Africa. Indigenous cultures have used them for centuries for spiritual and healing purposes (Guzmán, 2012).
   - **Effects:** Psilocybin induces visual and auditory hallucinations, alters perceptions of time and space, and fosters introspection, often leading to spiritual insight and emotional openness.
   - **Therapeutic Uses:** Research indicates potential benefits in treating depression, anxiety, PTSD, and addiction (Carhart-Harris et al., 2016). Psilocybin-assisted therapy typically involves guided sessions with therapists to support emotional processing and integration.

- **Precautions**: It should be used in a safe environment with experienced guides or therapists. Individuals with a history of psychosis or severe mental illness should avoid psilocybin due to the risk of exacerbating symptoms. It can interact with medications like SSRIs, MAOIs, and antipsychotics, so consulting a healthcare professional is essential.

2. **Ayahuasca:**
   - **Origin**: A psychoactive brew traditionally used by Indigenous tribes in the Amazon, made from the *Banisteriopsis caapi* vine and *Psychotria viridis* leaves (Tupper, 2008).
   - **Effects**: Ayahuasca induces intense visionary experiences, emotional purging, and deep introspection, often resulting in profound spiritual and emotional healing.
   - **Therapeutic Uses**: Used for treating depression, addiction, trauma, and existential distress, typically in ritualistic ceremonies guided by experienced shamans or facilitators (Labate and Cavnar, 2014).
   - **Precautions**: Should only be consumed in ceremonial settings under the guidance of experienced facilitators. It is contraindicated for those with cardiovascular issues or conditions like bipolar disorder or schizophrenia due to potential interactions with MAOIs.

3. **Ibogaine:**
   - **Origin**: Found in the root bark of the iboga plant, native to Central Africa, particularly Gabon, Cameroon, and Congo. Traditionally used in Bwiti ceremonies (Alper, 2001).
   - **Effects**: Produces intense, long-lasting psychedelic experiences with visual hallucinations and deep introspection, often facilitating addiction recovery.
   - **Therapeutic Uses**: Known for interrupting addictive patterns and promoting emotional processing and spiritual growth.
   - **Precautions**: Administration must be done by experienced providers due to potential serious side effects like cardiac

toxicity and seizures. Comprehensive medical screening and monitoring are crucial.

4. **Mescaline**:
   - **Origin**: Found in cacti like peyote, San Pedro, and Peruvian torch, used for centuries by Indigenous people in ceremonial practices (Smith, 2017).
   - **Effects**: Induces visual hallucinations, sensory perception changes, and introspection, typically lasting 8–12 hours.
   - **Therapeutic Uses**: Explored for treating depression, anxiety, PTSD, and addiction, mescaline can promote introspection and emotional processing.
   - **Precautions**: Should be used with caution in a supportive environment. Consult healthcare professionals if underlying mental health issues or medical conditions are present due to potential interactions.

5. **DMT (Dimethyltryptamine)**:
   - **Origin**: Naturally occurring in various plants and the active ingredient in ayahuasca (Strassman, 2001).
   - **Effects**: Induces short-lived, intense psychedelic experiences with visual and auditory hallucinations, often leading to spiritual insights.
   - **Therapeutic Uses**: Promotes spiritual insights, emotional healing, and personal growth.
   - **Precautions**: Best used in a safe environment with experienced guides. Those with severe mental illness or certain medical conditions should avoid it due to possible interactions.

6. **Bufo/Toad Medicine (5-MeO-DMT)**:
   - **Origin**: Derived from the venom of the *B. alvarius* toad, native to the Sonoran Desert.
   - **Effects**: Induces intense, short-lived psychedelic experiences characterized by ego dissolution and a sense of unity with the divine (Davis et al., 2019).
   - **Therapeutic Uses**: Facilitates emotional healing and spiritual insights and has shown potential in addressing various mental health concerns.

- **Precautions**: Should only be administered by experienced facilitators. Individuals with cardiovascular problems or mental health conditions, especially those taking specific medications, should avoid it due to potential interactions.

7. **Kambo**:
   - **Origin**: Derived from the secretions of the *Phyllomedusa bicolor* frog from the Amazon rainforest, used traditionally by some Indigenous tribes (den Brave et al., 2014).
   - **Effects**: Induces physiological effects like purging, increased heart rate, and sweating, which can promote physical detoxification.
   - **Therapeutic Uses**: Used for its purgative and cleansing properties, sometimes in treating depression, anxiety, addiction, and chronic pain.
   - **Precautions**: Should be administered by trained practitioners. Those with heart problems, high blood pressure, or epilepsy should avoid it due to potential risks.

Synthetic Psychedelic Drugs

8. **LSD (Lysergic Acid Diethylamide)**:
   - **Origin**: A synthetic compound derived from lysergic acid, first synthesized by Albert Hofmann in 1938 with its psychoactive effects discovered in 1943 when Hoffman ingested a dosage before a bicycle ride (Hofmann, 1980).
   - **Effects**: Produces visual and auditory hallucinations, altered perception of time and space, and profound introspection.
   - **Therapeutic Uses**: Studied for treating anxiety, depression, PTSD, and addiction, promoting mystical experiences and emotional healing (Gasser et al., 2014).
   - **Precautions**: Should be used in a controlled environment with experienced guides. Those with severe mental illness should avoid it due to potential interactions.

9. **MDMA (3,4-Methylenedioxymethamphetamine)**:
   - **Origin**: A synthetic compound originally developed as a pharmaceutical.

- **Effects**: Enhances empathy, emotional openness, and a sense of connection.
- **Therapeutic Uses**: Shows promise in treating PTSD, anxiety, depression, and relational difficulties (Mithoefer et al., 2019).
- **Precautions**: Should be used in a therapeutic setting with trained therapists. Avoid overheating and dehydration. Consult healthcare professionals for potential cardiovascular or psychiatric concerns.

10. **Ketamine**:
- **Origin**: A dissociative anesthetic used in medical settings.
- **Effects**: Produces sedation and dissociative experiences, promoting introspection and ego dissolution.
- **Therapeutic Uses**: Recognized for its rapid-acting antidepressant effects, particularly in treatment-resistant depression (Zarate et al., 2006).
- **Precautions**: Should be administered under medical supervision due to potential risks.

The psychedelic drugs listed here show potential for expanding consciousness and healing mental health issues. However, they should be approached with caution, respect, and proper guidance from trained professionals. Integration of psychedelic experiences, ongoing therapy, and support are crucial for maximizing therapeutic potential while minimizing risks.

There may be other medicines not listed here and you are invited to explore what their origins, contraindications, and precautions around them may be. Understanding their origins provides insight into their cultural and therapeutic significance.

Summary: Preparing for a Psychedelic Experience

In this module, we explored the critical steps to prepare for a psychedelic experience. Proper preparation can significantly influence the nature and outcome of the journey, particularly when using Psychedelics for healing purposes. These substances, often rooted in ancient Indigenous medicines, require respect and understanding. When we are able to properly prepare for an experience, we are creating safety which can support a more transformative journey.

Key Support Elements for Your Journey:

1. **Creating Set and Setting:**

   We discussed the importance of the psychological and environmental factors that influence a psychedelic experience. Ensuring a positive mindset and a safe, comfortable environment is vital for a transformative experience.

2. **Preparing with Art Therapy:**

   Art Therapy can be a valuable tool, helping individuals connect with their emotions, intentions, and fears. Creating visual representations can guide and support you throughout the journey. We began with an Art Therapy directive for setting an intention. This is key before preparing for a NOSC experience; however, you choose for this.

3. **Preparing with Journaling:**

   By developing a journaling practice, you are supporting the integration of the left and right brain hemispheres, just as art, meditation, and Psychedelics do as well. This can become a healthy exercise for reflection and you move through the stages of preparation and integration.

4. **Preparing with Meditation:**

   Meditation is crucial for regulating emotions and providing mental clarity. Establishing a regular practice helps reroute neurotransmitters in the brain, supporting quick focus and nervous system regulation. When we use meditation as a preparatory exercise for psychedelic therapy, we are developing a way to feel safe within NOSC experiences. Meditation connects you to a sense of Self that can easily feel lost when in the throes of a psychedelic experience. It helps to ground you when you may need it most.

5. **Dietary and Medication Precautions:**

   There are some foods, supplements, and medications that can interact with certain Psychedelics. This chapter gives an overview of the main ones to avoid to ensure safety and effectiveness.

Consulting healthcare professionals about current medications or supplements is essential.

6. **Avoiding and Managing Adverse Experiences:**

    Proper preparation helps minimize the risk of adverse experiences, or "bad trips." Strategies include engaging in positive mindset practices, choosing the right environment, ensuring physical well-being, and having a plan for managing challenging experiences. It is also important to establish what your plan is for integration before embarking on your journey.

7. **Serotonin Sickness:**

    The result of contraindicating medications or supplements mixing with certain Psychedelics. Serotonin sickness can be fatal, so it is important to know how to avoid and manage if this becomes a symptom.

8. **Different Psychoactive Drugs and their Origins:**

    Discussed in this model are the many different drugs used, their effects, origins, and what the difference is between synthetic Psychedelics and organic.

In summary, thorough preparation involving intention-setting, meditation, diet, and environmental factors are crucial for a safe, positive, and transformative psychedelic journey.

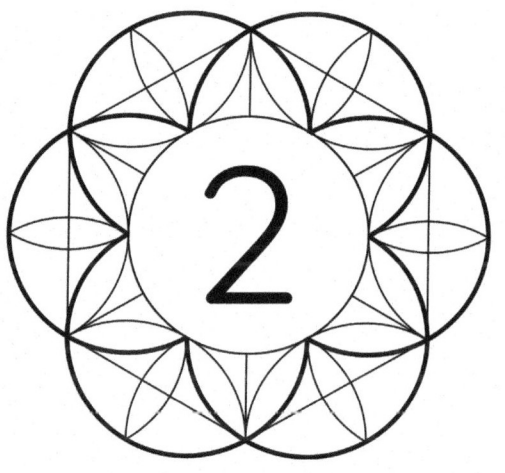

MODULE 2
THE IMPORTANCE OF GROUNDING AFTER PSYCHEDELICS

Rebuilding Your Aura after a Psychedelic Experience

In this module, there is a focus on coming 'back to earth' after your awakening experience. We will be working with a variety of somatic meditations, psycho-education, and specific Art Therapy directives to ground the non-ordinary experience you went through and solidify the healing benefits of this into your life.

Tapping into the somatic expression of your experience allows true and lasting transformation to take effect. Once identified, this is a tool you may use again and again to support you in life. As we pay attention to sensations in our body with mindful intent, we develop a relationship to the messages and wisdom it holds. By connecting the body, mind, and spirit, we bring a calmness back to ourselves that helps us to see the path that lies ahead on our journey of integration.

Non-ordinary states of consciousness, especially with powerful plant medicines and entheogens, have the effect of moving us emotionally and vibrationally from one state to another very quickly. This can take a toll on the energy force around the body that stabilizes and protects us from other people's energies, often referred to as our "aura." It is important to rebuild our auric strength after experiencing a non-ordinary state where we might have had the feeling of moving from one world to another so quickly.

DOI: 10.4324/9781003595762-21

The aura is the electromagnetic field that surrounds your body; it acts as a container for your life force. Like a shield, a strong aura attracts positivity and repels negativity. It gives a strong sense of security and an uplifting presence. A weak aura can allow negativity to penetrate the psyche and physical body, making you feel paranoid or lacking in self-trust.

This chapter focuses on rebuilding our aura by connecting to our breath, the present moment, nature, and feelings and sensations in the body. We will be using both meditation and art directives, to ground your energies and feel the sensations of the energetic field around you growing stronger and brighter. As we tap into the subtle energetic systems we are a part of, we build and strengthen the container we use to walk through this world.

Art Directive: Post Psychedelic Journey
What Your Experience Has Brought You

Materials Needed:

- Large piece of paper
- Writing/coloring tools: colored pencils, markers, crayons, pastels, pens, etc.
- Any additional materials that resonate with you

The purpose of this exercise is to take an inventory of your experience with psychedelic medicine, using creative expression as a means of processing. This directive helps ground your journey and integrate its insights into your present and future. Consider the following prompts:

1. How do you feel at this moment after your journey?
2. Reflect on how life was before your experience.
3. Where do you envision yourself going in the future, and what key takeaways will you carry forward?

As with any art-based activity, begin by centering yourself. Take a moment to notice your current physical state, connecting with your breath. Slowly inhale and exhale five times, focusing on deepening each breath.

By breathing into the belly, you activate the parasympathetic nervous system, promoting a state of relaxation (Porges, 2011). Feel your body being supported by the ground, chair, or surface you are on, pressing your feet into the floor to anchor your awareness.

As you relax further, become aware of any sensations in your body, be they physical or mental—acknowledge these sensations without judgment. The act of allowing them to arise and then gently pass with each breath helps you maintain a state of mindful presence (Kabat-Zinn, 1990). You may move your body in any way that feels right to release physical tension or discomfort.

Now, direct your attention inward, focusing on the solar plexus or heart area. This is where you will create from, tapping into your inner intuition and wisdom. Visualize drawing energy into this space. If you struggle to connect with this energy, imagine it being filled with light and strength as you breathe into it. By engaging with the heart center, you access a deeper unconscious process, as research suggests the heart has its own neural network, often referred to as the "heart–brain" (McCraty and Childre, 2010).

When you are ready, open your eyes and turn your focus to the art materials in front of you. You are invited to create a visual representation of your experience, highlighting where you were before, where you are now, and your hopes for the future. Use images, symbols, or drawings to express this journey rather than words, if possible. This allows you to engage the right hemisphere of your brain, which is more connected to emotions and intuition than analytical thinking (Malchiodi, 2003). However, if using words feels more comfortable, trust that intuition. Remember, the aim is to stay connected to the heart's energy rather than overthinking the process.

Scientific evidence indicates that when we create from the heart center, we access a more profound, unconscious space that can facilitate deeper understanding and transformation (McCraty and Childre, 2010). Engaging in art-making from this place can bring about a visceral shift in how we view and process our experiences.

As you create your map, take note of any emotions or thoughts that arise. Allow the process of moving feelings from within your body to the page to be a form of release and expression. This act of externalizing your experience can serve as a powerful tool for integration, helping to bring insights from your journey into conscious awareness.

After completing your art, spend some time journaling. Reflect on any thoughts or emotions that surfaced during the creative process and explore what your image communicates to you. Journaling in this way allows for further exploration and deepens the integration of your psychedelic experience (Franklin, 2017).

This exercise combines mindful self-awareness, creative expression, and the science of heart-centered processing to facilitate a deeper understanding of your journey, providing a foundation for lasting transformation.

Art Directive: Connecting to the Earth

Materials Needed

- Hot glue gun and hot glue sticks
- Various art materials: paintbrushes, glitter
- Ribbon, string, buttons
- Wood glue
- Natural materials (gathered outdoors) to create a representation of a safe, sacred space

Where Are You Now? Where Were You Before Your Ceremonial Experience?

- **Visualize a safe place:** Before beginning this art directive, take a moment to close your eyes and imagine yourself in a place in nature that feels safe and nurturing. This visualization helps ground your intentions for the exercise.

Walking Meditation Outside

Allow yourself to step outside into an area that feels comforting and nurturing. If possible, remove your shoes and socks to directly connect with the earth beneath your feet. As you begin to walk, take deep, full breaths of fresh air, focusing on the sensations beneath your feet with every step (Jones-Callahan, 2016). Walk slowly and with intention, allowing yourself to notice any objects in nature that capture your attention. This process aligns with nature-based mindfulness practices, which have been shown to reduce stress and promote a sense of well-being (Kabat-Zinn, 1990; Jordan and Hinds, 2016).

As you walk, mentally ask for permission from the earth to use these natural objects in your artwork. Continue for as long as you feel drawn to, staying connected to your breath and the ground beneath you. Walking meditation fosters mindfulness and a sense of presence, enhancing your connection to the earth and preparing you for the creative process (Kabat-Zinn, 1994).

Create Your Art

Return to your chosen sacred space and begin creating the artwork that comes to you. Gather the natural objects and art materials you feel drawn to, and allow the process to unfold organically. There are no rules here; this exercise is about the act of creation rather than the end product.

Focus on the process rather than the outcome. If you find your mind wandering toward planning or analyzing what you intend to make, gently shift your focus to the sensations in your body. Art Therapist Margaret Jones-Callahan (2016) emphasizes in her work, *Mindfulness Based Art*, that staying present in the creation process allows for a deeper exploration of inner thoughts and feelings, promoting a sense of grounding and self-discovery. Pay attention to changes in your breath and physical sensations as you work; this mindful awareness can help unlock inner wisdom and foster emotional release (Hinz, 2009).

Reflection

Once you have finished your creation, take some time to sit with it. Notice if there are any new sensations in your body now that you have completed the artwork. If it feels appropriate, ask your creation if it has any messages for you (Allione, 2008). This dialoguing process with art aligns with Jungian approaches to active imagination, where interacting with visual symbols can facilitate deeper insight and understanding (Jung, 1969c).

Finally, take some time to journal about your experience. Reflect on any thoughts, feelings, or bodily sensations that surfaced during and after the creative process. Journaling can help integrate the emotions and insights gained through art-making, further supporting your journey (Franklin, 2017).

This art directive encourages a deep connection with nature and self through mindful gathering and creative expression, helping you integrate your experiences in a grounded and meaningful way.

Narrative Therapy: Creating Your Self-Healing Routine

Write down everything you remember from your non-ordinary state, including your emotions immediately after the experience and the intention you set before you began the journey. Additionally, note any questions that have lingered for you since. Leave a few blank pages afterward to revisit and expand on any details or insights that arise as you continue to reflect.

Consider this part of your journal as a living document—a space to return to as you gain new awareness during this integration process. Giving this section a title page, perhaps with an art piece or simple doodles, can symbolize your ongoing commitment to this path of self-exploration and healing.

The goal of this work is to facilitate lasting healing from your experience. True integration occurs when you consciously apply the wisdom received during your journey to make meaningful life changes. This process helps create a solid foundation for your growth and transformation. While you may choose to engage in another psychedelic or mystical experience in the future for further self-reflection or consciousness expansion, it is essential to continually check in with your inner healer. By integrating your experiences thoughtfully, you strengthen and nurture your inner power (Polster and Polster, 1973).

When journaling, it is equally important to create a quiet, safe, and uninterrupted environment. Light candles, burn incense, or play calming music to help establish a personal, sacred space. This intentional atmosphere supports your inner wisdom as it flows onto the pages. Remember to breathe deeply; we often hold our breath while concentrating. A conscious breath can help move energy within you onto the page in front of you.

Understanding Neuroplasticity

The Power of Your Breath on Brain Health and Emotional Regulation

The breath is a powerful source of transformation. The rate and rhythm of the breath are intimately connected to our mental and emotional states

(Brown and Gerbarg, 2012). Just as emotions and the mind cause the breath to vary; by consciously controlling the breath, we gain control over our mind and our emotions (Trinity College Dublin, 2018a).

In my Art Therapy practice, one of the first things I pay attention to when I first see a client is how they are breathing. Noticing the breath says a lot about how a person is feeling at the moment. Notice how you are breathing right now. Is your breath shallow and regulated to the upper chest? Or is it deep and concentrated in the belly? How do you feel at this moment?

One way to stabilize yourself when feeling a sense of anxiety or stress (where the breath becomes shallow and centralized in the upper chest) is to stop and focus your attention on the breath filling the lower belly with deep inhales through the nose. Combine this method of breathing with the eye gaze by noticing ten things in the room and saying, mentally to yourself or aloud, their color and what they are, as well as pressing the feet into the floor. This will activate your parasympathetic nervous system and bring you into a feeling of calmness (Brantley et al., 2007).

On the other hand, when a person is feeling the depths of depression and despair, they may sigh a lot, almost as if with a sense of defeat. The breath here is usually more in the belly. To bring more prana, or life force, into the body, I recommend sitting up straight, lengthening the spine, and with an open mouth, breathing deep and forcefully into the upper chest.

This activates the sympathetic nervous system and creates a sense of alertness and aliveness (Levine and Frederick, 2005). Taking this one step further, I would invite the client to raise both arms above the head as they inhale, allowing the eye gaze to follow the hands while keeping the chin level (Assay et al., 1987a). Five to ten of these breaths and you will feel a tingling in the whole body, with the eye focus becoming clearer and a sense of elation.

So how and why does this happen? The respiratory system is one of the only major systems in the body that is usually involuntary, but which can also be voluntarily controlled (Levine and Frederick, 1997). Our heart also beats involuntarily but if we want to control it, slowing down our breath brings us into a state of calmness and relaxation. When we are able to control the breath, we are able to control the way we feel in the moment and develop a sense of control over stress levels.

Breath is the life force that keeps us going. Your rate of breathing and state of mind are inseparable. Using a full yogic breath or pranayama technique and especially adding mantra or chanting reprograms your whole cellular memory (Khalsa et al., 2024). By consciously directing the flow of our breath, not only are we transporting life force, vitamins, minerals, and glandular secretions to our vital organs, but we are also transforming the way we think and the way we feel.

For thousands of years, ancient wisdom from the East has exalted the virtues of breath-focused practices such as pranayama and meditation for their numerous cognitive benefits, including increased ability to focus, decreased mind wandering, improved arousal levels, more positive emotions, decreased emotional reactivity, among many other benefits (Immergut and Yates Culadasa, 2017). What did they know that we are just now scientifically validating?

A new study by researchers at Trinity College Institute of Neuroscience and the Global Brain Health Institute at Trinity, Dublin, explains for the first time the neurophysiological link between breathing, cognition, and emotion. The research shows that how we breathe directly affects the chemistry of our brains in a way that can enhance our attention and improve our brain health. It was found that the levels of a natural chemical messenger in the brain called noradrenaline are released when we are challenged, curious, exercised, focused, or emotionally aroused. If produced at the right levels, noradrenaline helps the brain grow new connections (Trinity College Dublin, 2018b).

Outlined here by PhD candidate at the Trinity College Institute of Neuroscience and lead author of the study, Michael Melnychuk:

> Practitioners of yoga have claimed for some 2,500 years that respiration influences the mind. In our study, we looked for a neurophysiological link that could help explain these claims by measuring breathing, reaction time, and brain activity in a small area in the brainstem called the locus coeruleus, where noradrenaline is made. Noradrenaline is an all-purpose action system in the brain. When we are stressed, we produce too much noradrenaline and we can't focus. When we feel sluggish, we produce too little and again, we can't focus. There is a sweet spot of noradrenaline in which our

emotions, thinking, and memory are much clearer. This study has shown that as you breathe in, locus coeruleus activity is increasing slightly, and as you breathe out it decreases. Put simply, this means that our attention is influenced by our breath and that it rises and falls with the cycle of respiration. It is possible that by focusing on and regulating your breathing, you can optimize your attention level and, likewise, by focusing on your attention level, your breathing becomes more synchronized.

(Melnychuk et al., 2018)

Ian Robertson, Co-Director of the Global Brain Health Institute at Trinity, and Principal Investigator of the study, added:

Yogis and Buddhist practitioners have long considered the breath an especially suitable object for meditation. It is believed that by observing the breath and regulating it in precise ways—a practice known as pranayama—changes in arousal, attention, and emotional control that can be of great benefit to the meditator are realized. Our research finds that there is evidence to support the view that there is a strong connection between breath-centered practices and a steadiness of mind.

(Robertson et al., 2018, cited in Melnychuk et al., 2018)

Even more exciting in this area of research was the potential impact breathwork and meditation may have on the aging of the brain. Ian Robertson went on to speculate:

Our findings could have particular implications for research into brain aging. Brains typically lose mass as they age, but less so in the brains of long-term meditators. More 'youthful' brains have a reduced risk of dementia and mindfulness meditation techniques actually strengthen brain networks. Our research offers one possible reason for this—using our breath to control one of the brain's natural chemical messengers, noradrenaline, which in the right 'dose' helps the brain grow new connections between cells. This study provides one more reason for everyone to boost the health of their brain using a whole range of activities ranging from aerobic exercise to mindfulness meditation.

(Robertson et al., 2018, cited in Melnychuk et al., 2018)

It is always exciting to witness when Eastern healing modalities are accepted as scientifically proven in our Western medical system. My personal feeling is that this mirrors our global understandings and acceptance of one another, a sharing of information rather than a fear that another's viewpoint (or position) will taint or somehow invalidate our own. I look forward to more research being done in the areas of mindfulness, meditation, yoga, and neuroscience to help heal and transform our brains and the way we engage in the world.

Understanding Our Dreams

Our dreams ultimately hold meaning that only we can determine for ourselves. While Carl Jung's discoveries highlight the existence of a collective consciousness—allowing us to connect with deep ideas, beliefs, archetypes, and universal truths—interpreting a dream is most effective when we first focus on what it means to us personally.

Below are two separate exercises to support you in interpreting your dreams. Once you have a dream recorded, you may begin. For the first exercise, it is best to have a written transcription of your dream rather than a voice recording.

Materials Needed

- Journal
- Colored pens/markers
- (Optional) recording device
- The notes app on your phone (can use talk-to-text)

Dream Yoga

1. Notice the words you wrote down to describe your dream. Are there specific ones that stand out?
2. Begin circling or highlighting every word that holds significance and record these on a separate page, leaving space after each for more notes.

3. Now, look at each word you wrote on that separate page. Beside each word, write a definition of what that word represents to you.
4. Once finished, read these definitions in sequence. This process allows you to understand and interpret your dream on a whole new level!
5. If you'd like, use this interpretation as an inspiration for creating art.

Although I've seen this method taught by various people, it was first brought to my attention by Swami Sivananda Radha in a book she wrote called *Realities of the Dreaming Mind: The Practice of Dream Yoga* (1990).

Art and Dreams: A Gestalt Approach

A powerful way to explore and interpret your dreams is through art and reflective practice (Carpendale, 2021). In this method, taught to me by founder and Professor Emeritus, Monica Carpendale from the Kutenai Art Therapy Institute, you create a visual representation of a significant moment from your dream. This doesn't need to be a polished piece of artwork; instead, it serves as a tangible representation of the dream content. When depicting people, it is helpful to sketch full figures rather than stick figures, as this can provide a more holistic view of the dream's elements (McNiff, 1992).

While creating, it is important to stay present with your body, paying close attention to any emotions that arise and maintaining awareness of your breath. Choose a serene, safe space to work—somewhere you feel comfortable and free from interruptions. Creating a calming atmosphere, perhaps by lighting candles or burning incense, can further support this reflective process.

Once your artwork is complete, examine all its components. Using an "I" statement, invite each part of the image to reveal its message. For instance, if you've drawn a figure standing by a window, ask it directly, "What message do you have for me?" Respond using "I am," "I have," or "I feel" to connect more deeply with the imagery (Carpendale, 2021). This self-dialogue is similar to the Gestalt therapy technique of giving voice to different aspects of the psyche, allowing unconscious feelings to surface (Polster and Polster, 1973). Stay grounded by breathing deeply into your belly and feeling the connection with the ground through your feet or seat. Listen for any responses that may emerge, such as "I am curious," "I am afraid," or "I want to be seen," and write them down, noticing the emotions these messages evoke.

You can extend this practice to inanimate objects in your dream, such as a door, table, or lamp. Engage with these objects in the same way, exploring their potential significance by asking them about their origins, roles, and needs. Write down any insights that come forward, maintaining an open, curious mindset throughout the process.

After completing your exploration, consider if there is anything in the image that requires change or adjustment. Are there elements that need transformation for healing or alignment? By making these changes directly in the artwork, you can symbolically address aspects of the dream, facilitating a deeper sense of integration and understanding (Rubin, 2010).

In this piece of reflection after a dream I had, I decided to use chalk pastels as they seemed to allow my image to be created quickly and felt

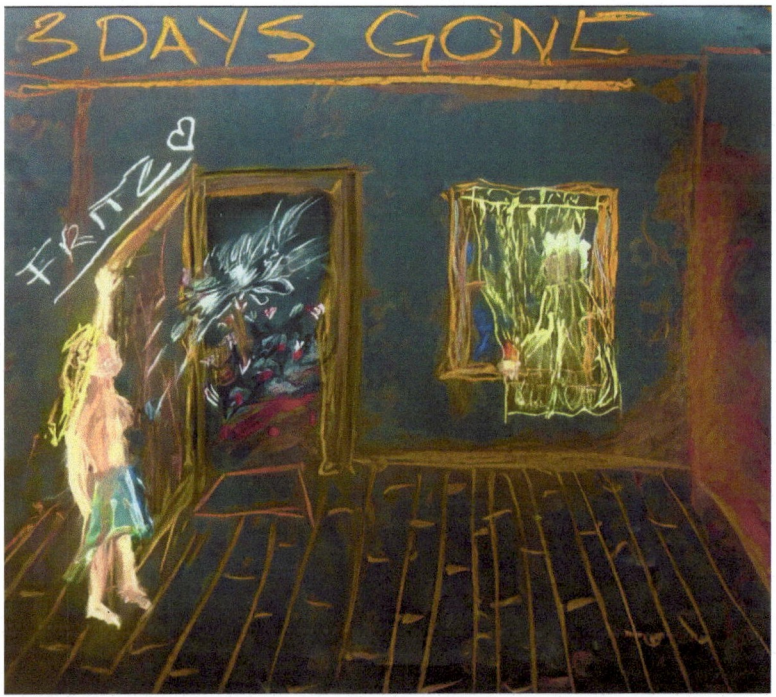

Figure 19.1 Understanding Our Dreams. An Example of Dream Art by Charmaine Husum, 2015

cathartic. It also felt significant to use black paper. I titled the image "3 Days Gone" since the theme of the dream was my cat going missing. I noted the feeling I had when I woke up: panic and emotional pain mixed with grief (my cat, Fritz, had passed away five years earlier).

I drew feverishly, getting out every aspect of the dream I could remember, with more details coming to light as I created. Staying connected to my breath and any feelings that emerged, I was feeling such deep sadness at Fritz's passing but knew the dream held far more meaning than that.

In order to access that information, after finishing the image, I began allowing each part of the art to speak with an "I" voice. I was surprised at what came out. I gave an "I" voice to the image of the woman standing at an open door. I also allowed the door frame to speak, the window that was open, the window frame, the curtains, the floor mat, the person outside of the window, the faintly drawn tree outside, and whatever it was that was coming in through the door. Finally, the dark room itself spoke, giving me even further insight into this dream.

I invite you to try this process for yourself, asking with non-judgmental curiosity what your unconscious would like to share with your waking mind.

Meditation for an Open Heart

Committing to a 40-day practice is a powerful support when changing our habits and life in general. I recommend this meditation to support you in that 40-day commitment.

For anyone experiencing stress, anxiety, or overwhelm with the constant stream of information that comes at us daily, this Meditation for an Open Heart can be extremely helpful. With consistent practice, you can come into a neutral, non-reactive place and feel steady and graceful amidst the turbulence that our world can sometimes create.

Practice this meditation to relieve yourself of anxiety, strengthen your immune system, open your heart, and bring clarity to your relationships. This meditation brings great stillness to the heart center and gives you space to perceive and assess your relationships from a more neutral place.

Note: Do not hold the breath in or out so long that you're gasping, in distress, or pressurizing the head. You may need to experiment a bit.

In my experience, holding the breath out is more difficult than holding the breath in. It can be frightening because there is no breath, and some even start to feel panicked. This is an opportunity to confront and move beyond fears while creating safety within.

Instructions

1. Sit in a comfortable posture with a straight spine and the chin slightly tucked to lengthen the back of the neck.
2. Either close the eyes or look straight ahead with the eyes 1/10th open.
3. Place the left hand on the center of the chest at the Heart Center. The palm is flat, pressed against the chest, with the fingers parallel to the ground, pointing to the right.
4. Make Gyan Mudra with the right hand (touch the tip of the index/Jupiter finger with the tip of the thumb). Raise the right hand up to the right side as if giving a pledge. The palm faces forward, and the three fingers not in Gyan Mudra point up.
5. The elbow is relaxed near the side with the forearm perpendicular to the ground.
6. Concentrate on the flow of the breath. Regulate each bit of the breath consciously.
7. Inhale slowly and deeply through both nostrils. Then suspend the breath in and raise the chest. Hold here as long as possible without pressurizing the head.
8. Exhale smoothly, gradually, and completely. When the breath is totally out, lock the breath out for as long as possible.

Eye focus:

- Either close your eyes and focus on the third eye point (between the eyebrows) or look straight ahead with your eyes 1/10th open.

To end:

1. Inhale and exhale strongly 3 times.
2. Relax.

Time:

- 3–31 minutes

How It Works

The entire posture induces a feeling of calmness. The left hand is for receiving and is placed at the heart center, creating deep stillness at that point. The right hand is for giving, for projecting, for throwing you into action and analysis. It is placed in a receptive, relaxed mudra and put in the position of peace.

Emotionally, this meditation adds a clear perception to your relationships with yourself and others. If you are upset at work or in a personal relationship, sit in this meditation for 3–5 minutes before deciding how to respond. Then act with your full heart.

Physically, this meditation strengthens the lungs and heart. It opens awareness of the breath, and it conditions the lungs. When you hold your breath in or out for "as long as possible," you should not gasp or be under strain when you let the breath move again.

Beginning a 40-Day Practice

Many of you may be familiar with the saying, "You are what you eat." But often, we may feel we have no control over what food is available to us. Or perhaps certain foods reward us even if we know they may not be good for us.

Another common saying is "Your habits define you." But when we feel we do not have control over those habits, how can we change them? Our habits become just that—habitual—and they begin to unconsciously control us instead of us consciously choosing them. Problems in life often originate from habitual behaviors that do not serve us but are unconsciously driving our actions.

In this practice of daily commitment, or "40-day practice," we use routine to consciously create control. You will be invited to commit to some form of practice that is available and accessible to you, with some options suggested.

As you read this instruction, notice how it makes you feel; is there excitement about doing something new and creating change, or is there resistance? Neither is good or bad. What is important is listening to the feelings that come up for you when you begin to explore your relationship with the things you do habitually in life. Our relationships with habits become entrenched in who we are, and releasing those that do not serve us can be a battle. There may be a sense that we need them to survive. There may even be comfort and familiarity with them, but what truly has control there? You or the habits?

Life can be said to be based on our habits—those things we do every day that all add up to who we are and how we walk in the world. Our habits define us to ourselves and to other people. They can give us a sense of control in our lives or a lack thereof. Habits can create peace and happiness in our world or misery and pain.

Accepting our habits without judgment becomes a large theme within this program. This is how we are able to attain love and acceptance of self in all its many facets of survival. Once we open a door to awareness and acceptance of the parts within us that hold habitual behavior, we can contemplate consciously choosing to create change in our lives. Although this can be challenging work, the benefits of making these changes can be transformative.

Within many world views and practices, committing to an ongoing routine for a specific amount of time helps to reroute habitual behavior, giving one a sense of control over their life. Below is an outline of some time blocks I learned through my teachings in yoga to alter habitual behaviors. You are invited to start with a 40-day practice if that is available to you and go from there as you choose.

You are welcome to use any of the meditations provided in this program for your commitment or choose one that you are already familiar with and that is personal to you.

Ancient yogic teachings believe that the number of days you can stick with a practice will affect your habits in different ways:

- 40 Days: Practicing every day for 40 days straight will support breaking any negative habits that block you from the expansion that is possible through meditation or mantra.
- 90 Days: Practicing every day for 90 days straight will establish a new habit in your conscious and subconscious mind based on the

effect of the meditation or mantra. You will notice a significant change.

- 120 Days: Practicing every day for 120 days straight will confirm the new habit of consciousness created by the meditation. The positive benefits of your practice become integrated permanently into your psyche.
- 1000 Days: Practicing every day for 1000 days straight will allow you to master your new habit of consciousness that the meditation or mantra has intended. No matter what the challenge, you can call on this new habit to serve you.

In this book, you have the opportunity to create lasting change in your life. As mentioned, you are encouraged to engage in any daily practice that serves and resonates with you. One recommended practice is a short and simple meditation introduced earlier in this module called 'Meditation for an Open Heart.' This easy meditation can be done in 1 minute, 3 minutes, 11 minutes, or hour-long increments. It will help balance your mind, body, and spirit, bringing you deep calmness and fostering profound love for yourself and those around you.

Summary: The Importance of Grounding after Psychedelics

In this module, we explored the essential steps to ground and rebuild your energy following a psychedelic experience. Proper grounding helps solidify the healing benefits and integrates the non-ordinary experiences into your daily life, ensuring lasting transformation. This involves self-care practices, including somatic meditations, psycho-education, and Art Therapy, to anchor the healing benefits of the experience into everyday life. By attentively tuning into the body's sensations and nurturing the connection between mind, body, and spirit, the path to lasting transformation and renewed calmness is paved.

Key Support Elements for Your Journey

1. **Rebuilding Your Aura After a Psychedelic Experience:**
    This module explores how non-ordinary states can affect the aura, the electromagnetic field that surrounds the body. These experiences can leave you vulnerable to the energies of those

around you and may destabilize your sense of Self. A strong aura attracts positivity and repels negativity, while a weak aura can lead to feelings of paranoia or a lack of self-trust. To rebuild auric strength, focus on connecting with your breath, staying present in the moment, engaging with nature, and tuning into your body sensations.

2. **Art Directive: Post Psychedelic Journey:**

    This exercise involves using large paper and various writing or coloring devices to reflect on your experience. It encourages taking an inventory of where you are now, where you were before, and where you hope to go. The process involves mindful breathing, connecting to the body, and creating a visual representation of your journey.

3. **Art Directive: Connecting to the Earth:**

    This exercise involves gathering natural materials and creating a representation of a safe, sacred space. It includes a walking meditation to connect with the earth, focusing on sensations beneath your feet, and creating art from collected natural objects to ground and support your energy.

4. **Narrative Therapy:**

    Immediately after a psychedelic journey, documenting your experience can help you remember and process what you've gone through. This introduction to a journaling practice is to encourage you to begin a regular routine of reflecting on your experiences during integration. This process will support you as you move through the various stages of integration outlined in this book, and provide deeper insights as you reflect on your creative expressions. Creating a living document allows for ongoing reflection and understanding, helping to deepen your integration journey.

5. **Understanding Neuroplasticity:**

    Using a psychoeducational lens, we explore here how the breath affects brain health and emotional regulation. Conscious breathing can influence the brain's chemistry, enhancing focus and emotional control. The research shows that breath-centered practices can have profound cognitive and emotional benefits.

6. **Understanding Our Dreams:**

    Exercises for interpreting dreams through writing and art are provided. These methods help unlock the subconscious messages in dreams, supporting deeper understanding and integration of non-ordinary experiences.

7. **Meditation to Open the Heart:**

    A specific meditation practice is introduced to support a 40-day commitment to grounding and relaxing the heart. This meditation helps manage stress, anxiety, and emotional turbulence, promoting a sense of peace and clarity. It is also the recommended meditation for your 40-day practice.

8. **Beginning a 40-Day Practice**:

    In this model, we discuss the importance of creating a routing with a meditation practice and ways that this routine will support you moving forward.

In summary, this module provides a detailed guide to grounding and rebuilding your energy after a psychedelic experience which is key in the first stage of integration. Here we lay the framework for the deeper processes that will be explored through the rest of this book. The suggested activities of somatic meditations, Art Therapy, breathwork, nature connection, and understanding dreams to integrate and solidify the healing benefits into your daily life are guides for your process however, altering these suggestions to fit your own path toward healing are always encouraged. Establishing nurturing habits builds a foundation of resilience and self-love. This compassionate journey supports ongoing personal growth, helping navigate life with renewed strength and clarity as you build a strong foundation for ongoing personal development and resilience after you NOSC experience.

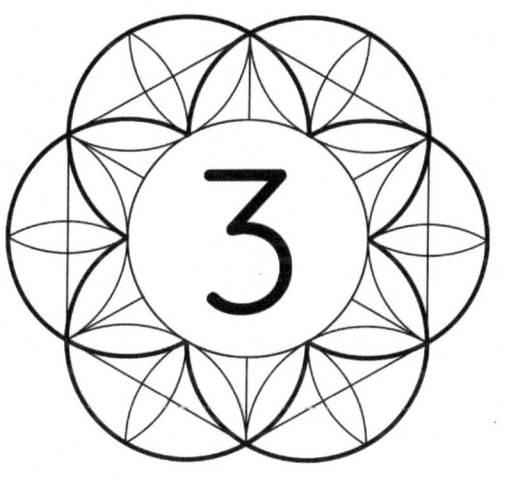

MODULE 3

CREATING SAFETY AND STRENGTHENING RESOURCES

Identifying Resources That Support You

As you continue this journey of integration, it's important to identify the strengths and resources you currently have in your life. There may be times during this healing process that feel difficult and even dismantling to your current life structure. For this reason, you may need to lean on the resources you have been identifying.

Take some time to journal about things in your life that bring you joy or a sense of control. This process invites a deeper sense of gratitude, which can support and sustain you. These might include time spent with a pet, family, friends, self-care practices, or even small things that you can control. Use these when you feel you need more support.

Another resource within your control is creating a routine, even in the smallest of things—something you can engage in every day. Examples include brushing your teeth, drinking a glass of water every morning or evening before bed, going to sleep and waking at the same time, going for a daily walk, journaling every evening before bed, or meditating daily. Choose something specific to you and what you feel is available and possible. It doesn't need to be a huge undertaking; allow yourself to start small with something manageable.

 DOI: 10.4324/9781003595762-22

There are many resources you can connect with. In this module, you will create a representation of a resource using art materials. You will also continue leaning into your daily meditation practice and recording your dreams to connect with the personal strengths inside that keep you going when you are feeling the stresses of life. As you focus on strengths and consciously map the progress you have made, you instill safety as you move through the journey of integration.

If your psychedelic or Non-Ordinary State of Consciousness (NOSC) experience felt supportive, the memory and energy of this can become one of your greatest resources on your journey through integration. For those who have used plant medicine, such as Ayahuasca or Psilocybin, there is a powerful spirit to these medicines that people have described being able to tap into, even years after their ceremony. There can also be a spirit or energy within experiences using synthetic Psychedelics or another means to achieve a NOSC. Remembering positive and transformative moments from your journey—however they were achieved—and expressing them through art or journaling can turn them into powerful allies on your path of integration.

If your psychedelic experience was difficult, consider whether there were aspects of it that brought release or awareness of parts inside that you had never examined before. Even though difficult, these pieces can be viewed as gifts that move you toward a deeper understanding of yourself, similar to the pain a seed experiences as it breaks through its husk to begin growing into a plant.

Another strength you may lean into is your personal relationship with Spirit or Source Energy, which can become heightened as you continue your meditations. Is there something or someone you believe in that feels larger than yourself? This could be what some call God, Source Energy, or Nature; it may also be the feeling of connecting to a loved one or a pet that has passed, or angels and other supportive etheric beings. Whatever feels true for you, tapping into these supports can be very healing.

Ultimately, the strength you want to cultivate, continue to grow, and develop a relationship with comes from within; it is not outside of yourself. Develop a relationship with the place inside you that has brought you here to this point and supported and sustained you in life so far. This intuitive knowing that you hold within will keep you safe, grounded, and strong on your path to integrating the healing that has taken place.

Art Directive: Connecting to Your Inner Strength
Somatically and Creatively Experiencing Your Inner Power

This art directive was inspired by my long-time teacher and supervisor, Millie Cumming. She introduced me to the concept of working with a resource image, which was based on the methods described by Joy Schaverien (1992).

Materials Needed:

- Round piece of thicker paper, 5"–10" in diameter: Watercolor paper works great! Using a regular size and shape of paper is fine as well.
- Various art materials: Oil and chalk pastels work very well, but any paints, crayons, or other bright art materials will do. Sparkles are always a nice touch as well! Check out the dollar store for great deals on materials.

In this directive, you are invited to pay attention to the subtle sensations in your body. Notice any discomfort or irritation and breathe into these places, creating expansion and a clearing. Imagine an energetic release with each exhale and anything not serving you being absorbed into the earth.

Allow yourself to sense a place inside where you feel well-being; where you feel all is well.

- Notice this area and breathe into it.
- Notice what happens in this area as you do so. Does it expand? Does it get brighter?
- See if you can direct the breath there, knowing that this is the seat of your intuitive knowingness. This is the place inside that keeps you safe and loved always. The wisdom of your Soul lives here.

As you develop a connection and relationship with this area, see if you can visualize any colors that surround it or what it is made of. Is there a texture, a shape, or a felt sense of what it is? Breathe into this visualization, feeling complete calmness growing out of this area as it expands to include your whole being.

Now, after being with this space within you, ask if there are any messages it has for you. Stay open to any sensations or words that pop up and feel gratitude for this connection you have with your inner self. This is your own intuitive knowing that will always look out for you and hold the greatest good for your Soul's intent.

As you begin to come back into the room, take the round piece of paper and any art materials you have and begin to create a representation of what you saw within. This does not need to be an exact replica but something that will remind you of this place you hold within, an expression of what you saw. Allow yourself to feel this creation fully as you make it, staying connected to deep breathing and feeling yourself connected to the ground.

Use this creation as a reminder of your inner strength and put it up somewhere visible and near to you as you continue on your path to integration. The image you have created can become somewhat of a talisman (Schaverien, 1992), a resource object to refer to when moving into more difficult arenas of healing throughout this book.

Art Directive: Who or What Helps You Feel Supported?
Creating a 3-D Representation of Support

Materials Needed:

- Hot glue gun and hot glue sticks
- Various art materials: paint brushes, glitter
- Ribbon, string, yarn, buttons
- Wood glue
- Natural materials
- Fabrics of your choice
- Beads, ribbons, shells, buttons, or other miscellaneous objects that feel significant
- Clay or plasticine (optional)

In this Art Directive, you will create a 3-D object representing what supports you and makes you feel safe, loved, and connected. This could take the form of a doll, a person, an animal, or even an abstract creation that holds meaning for you.

If you are doing this by yourself or with a client, we recommend setting aside a quiet space where you will be uninterrupted if this is available to you. Play some relaxing music, light candles, and burn incense—whatever you may need to create a sacred space for yourself to feel deeply and explore using the materials.

It is also advised to begin your creative process after the yoga or meditation exercises offered in this module, to feel fully relaxed, tapping into the subtle sensations within your body. Yoga and meditation will shift your brain waves into a state that allows for deeper reflection and creative exploration.

Allow yourself to be moved by the materials instead of imagining in your mind what you want to make. Allow for fluidity in your creation. Notice the pieces or parts that may not work out the way you intend or may not stick, and breathe into the feelings that arise from that, knowing that everything is in perfect order and alignment. Trust the process and know that whatever comes up for you is meant to be expressed. There are no mistakes. Everything that happens in this space of creation is meant to happen for you to create and connect with the representation of what supports you.

In life, we are often unaware of the things that make us feel supported. They can pop up out of nowhere when we need them most. Hold this wonder in your heart as you allow yourself to be moved by the materials and to create unencumbered. Stay connected to your breath as you keep an awareness of the energy moving through you.

How Breathing Patterns Affect Your Nervous System
Instantly Regulate Emotions with Breath

1. **Notice Your Breath**
   - Observe your breath in this moment. Is it shallow or deep? Do you feel it filling your stomach or your chest?
   - Just be with your breath, noticing how you are breathing. This is your life force, called Prana.

Parasympathetic Engagement

2. **Belly Breathing:** When we breathe fully into our belly, we engage the parasympathetic nervous system, which helps bring on a sense of calmness.

   - Begin to lengthen your breath; close your eyes if that feels comfortable; slow your breath and feel each moment as you inhale fully.
   - Place your hand on your belly, holding yourself, feeling comforted.
   - Allow the breath to fill your belly first, then move into the lungs up to the clavicle. Pause, then release from the lungs, finally expelling all the breath from the belly by pushing it out. Repeat for 5 breaths.
   - Notice any body sensations that have arisen. Just be with these, observing and feeling a sense of relaxation, surrender, and release.
   - Try taking at least 5 of these full, expansive belly breaths.
   - This engages your parasympathetic system; notice the subtle feelings this breath brings to your body and mind.

Sympathetic System Engagement

3. **Chest Breathing:** As we shift the breath into our chest, we activate the sympathetic nervous system, which supports us in feeling alert, awake, and on guard.

   - Take 5 full breaths now and as you do, raise your arms above your head with eyes open, following your hands with your gaze as you raise them. Breathe fast and deeply into the upper chest.
   - Notice how you feel.
   - This engages your sympathetic system, helping you feel alert and present.
   - Now return your breath to normal and just notice where it goes, what feels most comfortable and familiar to you. Is it in the upper chest or the belly? What system are you currently engaging?
   - Take notice of this throughout this program and in your daily life.

Control through Breath:

By knowing ways to shift our nervous system through the use of breath, we gain a greater sense of control over our bodies (Brown and Gerbarg, 2012).

- If we are feeling depressed and down, there can be an overactivation of the parasympathetic system, often accompanied by large sighs and a sense of despair and hopelessness. Engaging in sympathetic nervous system breathing, such as quicker, more vigorous breaths, can help shift these feelings in the moment (Melnychuk et al., 2018).
- Conversely, when we are in an anxious state with a racing heart and a sense of panic, focusing our breath on the belly with full, slow breaths can help reduce the overactivation of the sympathetic nervous system, bringing us into a calmer state (Kabat-Zinn, 1990).

Meditation for Balancing the Brain's Hemispheres
Alternate Nostril Breathing (Nadi Shodhana Pranayama)

This practice originates from the ancient Indian tradition of Yoga (Saraswati, 1984). Nadi Shodhana is a Sanskrit term where "Nadi" means "channel" or "flow" and "Shodhana" means "purification." It is a technique used in pranayama (yogic breathing practices) to purify the nadis, which are the energy channels in the body, and to balance the flow of breath through the left and right nostrils (Feuerstein, 2001).

As you engage in this meditative breathing practice, focus on keeping your breath slow, smooth, and continuous. Focusing on your breath will help you stay present in the cycle. You want to breathe easily throughout the practice, so keep tissues close by if needed to clear your nasal passages.

To Practice Alternate Nostril Breathing:

In this pranayama, the breath is always relaxed, deep, and full (Brown and Gerbarg, 2012).

1. Sit in a comfortable position with your legs crossed (or with feet on the ground if seated in a chair), and keep your chin slightly pulled in to lengthen the back of the neck.

2. Place your left hand in Gyan Mudra, touching the index finger to the thumb, and rest it on your left knee. This mudra helps to focus the mind.

Throughout the meditation, use the thumb of your right hand to close the right nostril, and the index or ring finger of your right hand to close the left nostril.

1. Close your right nostril and gently inhale fully through your left nostril.
2. Then close your left nostril and exhale through the right.
3. Inhale through the right nostril.
4. Close the right nostril and exhale through the left.
5. Inhale through the left nostril.
6. Continue alternating nostrils after each inhalation.
7. Complete the practice by finishing with an exhale on the left side.
8. Continue for 11 minutes.

Benefits of Alternate Nostril Breathing:
- Promotes whole-brain functioning by balancing the right and left hemispheres (McCraty and Childre, 2010).
- Is both integrating and grounding.
- Purifies the body and mind.
- Creates a deep sense of well-being and harmony on the physical, mental, and emotional levels.
- Helps alleviate headaches, migraines, and other stress-related symptoms (Brown and Gerbarg, 2012).
- Inhale left, exhale right: Calms and integrates unwanted negative emotions and stress. Excellent before bed.
- Inhale right, exhale left: Enhances clarity and fosters a positive mood, helping with focus.

Breathing through the Left Nostril Is Associated With:

- Ida nadi, the energy point ending at the left nostril (Saraswati, 1984).
- Apana, the energy of cleansing and elimination.
- Moon energy: cooling, receptive, calmness, empathy, and sensitivity.
- Feminine energy that is warm, nurturing, and receptive.

Breathing through the Right Nostril Is Associated With:

- Pingala nadi, the energy point ending at the right nostril.
- Prana, the nurturing and vital energy.
- Sun energy: warmth, alertness, readiness-for-action, and willpower.
- Masculine energy that is direct, strong, and invigorating (Feuerstein, 2001).

Journaling and Reflections

Continuing Your Relationship with the Medicine and Art

As you move through each art directive and meditation in this journey, continue supporting your process by journaling your thoughts and feelings. Journaling is an effective tool for self-awareness, as it allows you to reflect on the meanings behind the symbols and elements in your artwork (Malchiodi, 2015). Pay attention to the sensations that arise in your body as you engage with the artwork. Breathe into those sensations, and connect with what supports you during this process. Allow your intuition to deepen, staying open to the messages that come to the surface.

A helpful technique for journaling is to ask your artwork if it has any messages for you. Sit calmly, wait, and see if anything arises in your mind or heart (Levine and Frederick, 1997). Write down any insights that come. If you'd like, continue the dialogue to connect more deeply with your intuitive knowing.

Take some time to reflect on how your non-ordinary experiences have been integrating so far. Ask yourself: Have any changes occurred? What are they, and how are they affecting your life? What thoughts or memories from the experience stand out? Use your journal as a space to allow these reflections to unfold, giving yourself time for deeper awareness and processing (Grof, 1997).

Another helpful method is to write out lingering questions. Start by writing your question in one color pen, take a moment to tune in to any internal guidance, and when you feel ready, write your answers using a different color pen. This technique has been known to foster a deeper connection with your inner guidance and intuition (Siegel, 2010a). You can also use this process to connect with other energies—like spirit guides, angels, or the medicine itself—depending on what resonates with you.

Precautions

Before opening yourself to non-physical energies, such as the spirit of the medicine, it's important to ensure you are protected. Ask only for the highest benevolent wisdom to show itself. A helpful practice is to burn sage or sweetgrass and set an intention or prayer, visualizing yourself surrounded by a bright white light (Kirmayer, 2004). Find what works best for you to create safety, both physically and energetically.

Working with entheogens opens a door to the spirit world. Once opened, it's crucial to practice energetic hygiene to ensure you're connecting only with positive, supportive energies (Grof, 2008b). This practice not only helps protect you but also strengthens your connection with your own intuitive wisdom and guidance.

Dreamwork

Art and Reflection for Deeper Meaning

As you move through the second module of this program, you are encouraged to reflect back to your dream journal, noticing any themes that may be emerging. Spend time now to read through your dreams. If you would like to expand further and gain more information about the subconscious processes happening for you in the dream state, refer back to page 33 to support you in your exploration.

You may also take an inventory at this point by journaling about themes you are noticing in your dreams. How are you feeling upon waking? Are you exhausted still or well-rested? Are there any emotions you feel as you wake? Allow your process of reflection and inquiry to be open with a non-judgmental curiosity.

Continuing Your 40-Day Practice

You have already moved into the third module of this book and hopefully had some time to begin your 40-day practice. If you have not yet begun, it is recommended to give it a try, even if it's just one minute a day. Do something in a quiet state of meditation and reflection that will support you. Whatever works for you. If you forget a day, that is fine, come back to it as soon as you remember.

If you have already begun, notice any shifts or changes in the way you are in the world. How are you feeling? How are you reacting to others? How has your mood been? Keep notice of the changes that are beginning and continuing to form. This will be of great support as we move through this program.

If you found the first Meditation for an Open Heart supportive from page 134, refer back to this as a regular practice. Otherwise, choose another from the meditations offered within this book or a favorite you already use.

Summary: Creating Safety and Strengthening Resources

In this module, we explored the crucial steps to identify and strengthen the resources that support you during the integration process after a psychedelic experience. Recognizing and cultivating the strengths and resources in your life is crucial for navigating this healing journey and will provide stability and resilience, especially during challenging times.

Key Support Elements for Your Journey:

1. **Connecting to Resources:** This module encourages processes to identify and get to know your resources. Engaging in art, daily meditation, and recording dreams connects you with your inner strengths and instills a sense of safety. One resource that you may want to connect to could be the energy of your experience or the spirit of the medicine. If your psychedelic or NOSC experience was supportive, these memories can serve as powerful resources

during integration. Expressing these moments through art or journaling can also be a significant ally in this process.

2. **Establishing Routine:** Create simple daily routines that are manageable and provide a sense of stability. Journal about what brings you joy and a sense of control. This practice fosters gratitude and sustains you, whether it involves time with pets, family, friends, self-care practices, or small daily routines. Establishing manageable routines, like brushing your teeth or going for a daily walk, provides stability and support.

3. **Art Directive: Who or What Helps You Feel Supported:** Here you are invited to create a 3-D object representing what makes you feel safe and connected. As you explore and express this support using various materials, you are encouraged to deepen your understanding of what sustains you.

4. **Art Directive: Connecting to Your Inner Strength:** This directive involves a meditation and the opportunity to create a visual representation of your inner strength using a round piece of paper and various art materials. The exercise focuses on paying attention to subtle body sensations and visualizing your inner power. As one of the most important somatic art directives within this book, the art you create here can be used as a resource image or talisman as we move into more difficult aspects of integration to help remind you of your inner strength and sense of self-energy. This art directive can also be a great one to use in preparation of your NOSC experience.

5. **Breathing Patterns and Nervous System Regulation:** Learn how different breathing patterns affect your nervous system. This experiential exercise offers an opportunity to shift nervous system engagement, moving from an activated sympathetic state to a relaxed parasympathetic state. Belly breathing engages the parasympathetic system for calmness, while chest breathing activates the sympathetic system for alertness. Understanding these techniques provides control over your emotional states.

6. **Meditation for Balancing the Brain's Hemispheres:** An ancient yogic breathing practice, alternate nostril breathing helps to

balance the brain's hemispheres, purify the body and mind, and create a sense of well-being and harmony.

7. **Dreamwork:** You are encouraged to continue reflecting on dream themes and record any insights in your journal. This practice uncovers subconscious processes and supports deeper understanding and integration. We use the dream state as another altered state to gain deeper awareness as we continue through the process of lasting healing after an NOSC.

8. **Journaling and Reflections:** Continue to journal about your thoughts, feelings, and insights, from meditations and art making. Use your art as a tool for reflection and dialogue with your inner guidance. This practice deepens your connection to intuition and supports ongoing integration.

9. **Precautions:** When working with altered states of consciousness, we are tapping into and opening up the spirit world. When connecting with non-physical beings or energies like the spirit of medicine, it's important to call on protection that only those supporting our greatest good be shown. Practice energetic hygiene to maintain positive connections and support your intuitive guidance. Ultimately, the strength you need comes from within. Develop a relationship with your inner self, the intuitive knowing that has guided you this far. This connection keeps you safe, grounded, and strong.

10. **Continuing Your 40-Day Practice:** Engage in your 40-day practice, even if it's just a brief daily meditation or reflection. Reflect on your progress noticing any changes in your feelings, reactions, and mood. Consistency in this practice can be very helpful as it supports your ongoing growth and integration.

Module Three emphasizes creating safety and strengthening resources to navigate your integration process effectively. This module follows the second stage of trauma therapy outlined in the protocols developed by Judith Herman (1992). By identifying and utilizing personal strengths, connecting with spiritual supports, and engaging in reflective practices, you foster resilience and sustain your healing journey through the integration process.

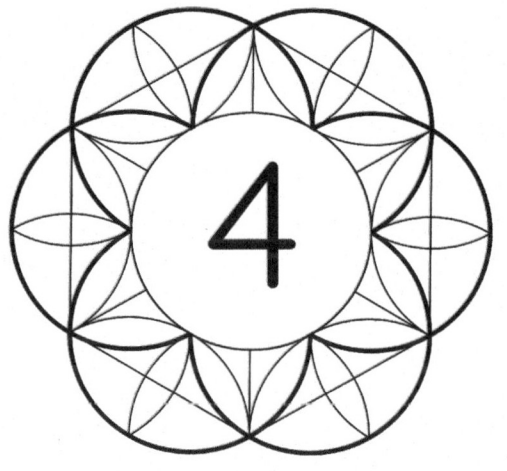

MODULE 4

CONNECTING TO THE SPIRIT OF THE EXPERIENCE

Working beyond the Transpersonal

Integrating the Tools Learned through Psychedelics

Long after experiencing a non-ordinary state of consciousness—whether through meditation, breathwork, or using entheogenic plant medicines—the energy and impact of that encounter often persist. For those who have journeyed with Ayahuasca, for example, many speak of the plant's spirit continuing to remain with them (Labate and Cavnar, 2014). In various Indigenous and Shamanic teachings, Elders describe certain plants as holding a lasting energy and power that stays with the person who has ingested them, whether the plant is psychotropic or not (Tupper, 2009). If this resonates with you, consider continuing this relationship by recognizing the plant's spirit as a guide for your ongoing healing. Developing and sustaining a long-standing relationship with plant medicines has been reported as a great support for many people (Fadiman, 2011).

Even if your experience was not plant-based, but instead arose from synthetic Psychedelics, deep meditation, or Kundalini awakening, you can still access the energy of that transformative moment. When the constructed sense of physical reality dissolves, insights often emerge that can be integrated into your body as visceral memories. Solidifying these memories can provide ongoing resources and support throughout your

DOI: 10.4324/9781003595762-23

integration process. Whether you believe the source of these experiences is external, such as Spirit or Source Energy, or internal, it remains beneficial to regularly access the memory and energy of that moment as a valuable resource (Winkelman, 2010).

In your meditations and art-making practices, take time to recognize both the wisdom gained and the path that led you to these insights. Strengthening this relationship to your journey fosters a deeper connection to yourself and increases self-trust. Similar to remembering a dream, the more you actively recall your experiences, the less likely you are to forget them, allowing for more effective integration of the knowledge gained (Grof, 1997).

I find that calling upon the spirit of the plants I have dieted, alongside my guides and angels, provides additional support. You may discover that through this practice, your mystical experiences become more deeply integrated into your daily life, benefiting you long into the future (Forte, 1997).

Integrating in this way aligns with a harm-reduction approach to healing. One potential challenge to watch out for is the tendency to seek out mystical experiences or non-ordinary states repeatedly. As we integrate, it's essential to focus on developing inner awareness and strength, so that healing is experienced internally, rather than as something we constantly seek externally. While Psychedelics themselves are not typically addictive, the desire for heightened experiences can be. Like any medicine, Psychedelics are tools for healing and should not be overused. It is essential to integrate your experiences fully so that you may reap the long-term benefits without over-relying on external sources for transformation (Marlatt, 1996).

Art Directive: Taking an Inventory of Your Life

Reflecting On Our Past, Present and Future

This directive has been adapted from that described in Monica Carpendale's book, *Essence and Praxis in the Art Therapy Studio* (2009). A precaution though that this directive may bring up past experiences that are triggering. Be mindful to take care of yourself before beginning so you feel resourced and only engage in memories you feel ready to explore. Using and observer's lens instead of going into the feelings can be helpful.

Materials Needed:

- Scissors
- Collage images
- Pencil crayons/markers (optional)
- Glue stick
- Beads, sparkles, natural materials, or other miscellaneous objects (optional)
- Bristol board or large paper (or a series of papers stuck together to create a longer, linear representation)

Before you begin this directive, create a sacred space where you will not be disturbed, allowing yourself to fully explore your personal timeline. In this space, include items or images that evoke a sense of security and joy. You may want to bring in the doll or totem you created in the last art directive, light candles, or play your favorite music. A brief meditation beforehand can help you feel grounded (Brown and Gerbarg, 2012), especially since this directive has the potential to evoke deep and powerful emotions.

In this directive, you will reflect on your life from the past to the present, leaving space for the future.

When thinking about the story of your life, you might be reminded of pivotal moments. These can be supportive memories or more challenging ones that had a significant impact. As you reflect on these moments, allow yourself to feel the impact, while staying grounded in the present. Let these emotions arise, move through you, and pass (van der Kolk, 2014).

It's common for painful memories, especially those connected to trauma, to feel as though they are happening in the present. When this happens, gently remind yourself that you are safe, loved, and protected right now—you are simply remembering (Herman, 1992).

To Begin:

1. Spend some time gathering images that represent pivotal moments in your life. You can do this during the directive or prepare by collecting images over time. If there is a specific image you want, you can print it from the internet or draw it in whatever way feels right.

2. Your timeline can start at any age and extend as far into the future as you like. If you place images in the future section, imagine these moments as real, keeping an open and grateful heart for what you want to manifest (Levine and Frederick, 1997).

3. You can arrange your images in a linear format by connecting pages together or using a large Bristol board (thicker poster-size paper), or can represent the past, present, and future in any way that feels right to you. If you feel more called to draw images into areas, do that. Or accentuate different areas with materials like beads or sparkles to bring emphasis to specific moments.

4. Notice the areas on your timeline when you have felt profound mystical shifts and experiences and spend time feeling these again in your body as you remember them. Close your eyes and breathe into these memories, do any feelings or sensations in the body come up? What area in the body do you feel it? What does it feel like? Take a moment to breathe into this area and if this feels positive and supportive, allow that feeling to spread throughout your body as you take full breaths inhaling and exhaling. If they are not supportive, use your breath to release them into the earth to be transformed into something resourceful (McEvoy and Ziegler, 2006).

5. Reflect on how your mystical experiences have influenced your timeline. Have any parts of your past, present, or future changed as a result? Draw connections between these shifts and your experiences.

6. Notice areas on your timeline that do not feel positive or supportive. Is there something you would like to change or add to these images and memories? Maybe ask them, "What were you trying to teach me?" and notice if you feel a visceral response in the body or an answer to your question that arises in another way.

7. Know that you are in a safe space now. It is safe to explore any memories that you feel ready to process. Stay connected to your inner power and the healing you've experienced from your mystical journey.

8. If you feel called, consider adding something resourceful to difficult memories on your timeline. For example, if a memory from your childhood needed more support, add an image of something

protective, like a teddy bear. For adult memories, consider adding an image of a hug or another comforting gesture. Stay connected to your body through your breath, tracking any sensations or shifts that occur.

Journaling after the Art

Once you've completed your timeline, take some time to process it. Begin journaling about any feelings or insights that have arisen. This is your process, so take this time to explore, ask questions, and make sense of the memories. Most importantly, remind yourself that you are in control of your life. Connect with the support available to you, whether from the spirit you encountered in your mystical experience or from within yourself (Assay et al., 1987).

Spiritual, Ineffable, and Etheric Aspects of the Psychedelic Journey

Psychedelic medicines often facilitate experiences that yield profound insights and altered perspectives, which can be life-changing. These substances act as catalysts, propelling individuals on deep internal journeys that challenge and expand their understanding of themselves and the universe. Many describe these experiences as mystical, providing new insights about how they engage with the world and others. Some of the most common insights observed, both personally and in clients, include:

A Deeper Sense of Belonging

Psychedelic experiences often cultivate a deep sense of interconnectedness, not just socially but universally. People frequently feel as if they are part of a greater whole, which can bring immense reassurance, particularly in a world often marked by isolation and disconnection (Watts et al., 2017). The effectiveness of Psychedelics in treating treatment-resistant depression may be linked to this newfound sense of belonging and interconnectedness (Carhart-Harris and Goodwin, 2017).

Purpose and Meaning

Psychedelics tend to prompt existential contemplation, stirring thoughts about life's big questions. By altering consciousness and presenting experiences that feel profoundly significant, these substances help individuals discover a sense of purpose aligned with their values and passions. This connection to meaning is critical for making transformative changes in daily life (Griffiths et al., 2008). Integration practices are essential to transferring these insights into sustained, purposeful living.

Understanding One's Place in the World

During psychedelic experiences, individuals often perceive layers of reality previously unseen. This shift in perspective can result in new understandings of their role in the world, prompting thoughts about their contributions and the legacy they wish to leave (Pollan, 2018).

Recognition of Life's Preciousness

Psychedelics can enhance appreciation for the preciousness of life. Experiences that make every moment feel rich with significance often lead individuals to return with a renewed zest for life and a stronger desire to make the most of their time on Earth (Ross et al., 2016). This shift in mindset, rooted in gratitude and appreciation for the world around us, is transformative in many people's lives.

Empathy and Moral Development

Psychedelic experiences can dissolve the boundaries between "self" and "other," increasing empathy. People may become more attuned to the feelings of others, fostering greater moral development and engagement with social or environmental causes. This enhanced empathy also reflects inwardly, promoting self-compassion, a critical area of struggle for many individuals (Michaels et al., 2018).

Renewed Spirituality

Even those who do not subscribe to traditional religious beliefs often emerge with a renewed sense of spirituality after using Psychedelics. This newfound spirituality is typically more personal and experiential, free from institutional religious structures, and often involves a deep connection to nature or a broader cosmic consciousness (Grof, 2008b). This connection to something larger provides greater safety and security in navigating the challenges of everyday life.

Integration of Shadow Self

Psychedelics have the unique ability to reveal repressed or unconscious parts of the psyche—what Carl Jung referred to as the "Shadow Self." Integrating these shadow aspects can result in deeper self-understanding and authenticity in one's life (Jung, 1969c). This crucial process will be explored further in Module Eight.

Coping with Mortality

Experiences of ego dissolution and encounters with the divine can profoundly alter one's perspective on death. By confronting mortality within a transcendent context, individuals may find comfort and diminish their fear of death, which significantly impacts how they choose to live their lives (Griffiths et al., 2016). Practitioners specializing in Palliative or End-of-Life care often work with Psychedelics to help individuals transition more peacefully through the process of dying.

Collective Unconscious

Some report accessing the collective unconscious during psychedelic experiences—a reservoir of shared memories and archetypes among all humans. Tapping into this shared humanity can cultivate a sense of unity and compassion that transcends individual or cultural differences (Winkelman, 2010).

Integrating these experiences into everyday life is critical for lasting benefit. A transpersonal approach to integration, which honors the spiritual and ineffable aspects of these journeys, can support individuals in applying their newfound insights and maintaining the sense of connection and purpose uncovered during the psychedelic experience (Grof, 2015).

Stanislav Grof: The Grandfather of Psychedelic Therapy

Stanislav Grof's ground-breaking work with LSD (Lysergic Acid Diethylamide) therapy illuminated the deeper layers of the unconscious mind that patients could access beyond addressing biographical and perinatal issues. His research revealed that psychedelic therapy often led to transpersonal experiences—states that transcend the individual ego, time, space, and personal history. These experiences include phenomena such as out-of-body experiences, past-life memories, ancestral memories, extrasensory perceptions, and remote viewing (Grof, 2000). For many who have undergone these experiences, they hold profound and authentic significance, even though they challenge conventional Western scientific models of the mind.

Grof suggested that the roots of some psychological problems might lie in these transpersonal realms. Whereas biographical experiences align with Freudian theories, transpersonal experiences resonate with Jung's concept of the collective unconscious. This opens up significant therapeutic potential, often leading to profound resolutions of deeply ingrained psychological issues during LSD therapy sessions (Grof, 1985). This aspect of Grof's work emphasizes how healing can occur in ways that transcend traditional therapeutic approaches, offering new pathways for addressing trauma and psychological blocks.

What fascinated Grof was the ability of patients under LSD to recount vivid, detailed past-life memories, sometimes with remarkable historical accuracy that they had no prior knowledge of. These revelations support Grof's theory that the unconscious mind holds vast, untapped dimensions of knowledge and experience, which can emerge during psychedelic therapy (Grof, 2008a).

Central to Grof's approach was the belief in the "Inner Healer"—the idea that within each individual lies an inherent capacity for healing, which can be unlocked and accessed during altered states of consciousness. This concept remains integral in the training for psychedelic-assisted therapies today, whether it involves MDMA, psilocybin, or other psychedelic medicines (Grof, 1993). Grof emphasized that the role of the therapist is not to guide the journey but to provide a safe and supportive environment, allowing the patient's inner wisdom to guide the healing process. This patient-led journey sometimes intensifies symptoms before they improve, further underscoring the importance of the therapist's role in offering non-directive support during these transformative experiences (Grof, 1976).

Meditation: Six Steps of Focusing

Getting to the Root of a Problem

The meditation and therapy technique I often use with clients to get to the root of a problem is based on the modality of "Focusing," developed by Eugene Gendlin and published in 1978. This approach helps clients discover an inner solution or "aha moment" that creates a noticeable shift in awareness around a particular issue. Focusing emphasizes identifying inner bodily sensations, also referred to as the "felt sense," which allows individuals to move beyond habitual patterns and gain clarity.

Gendlin's research demonstrated that a client's ability to experience lasting positive change in psychotherapy depends largely on their capacity to access this nonverbal, bodily awareness of the issues that brought them into therapy (Gendlin, 1978). By tuning into these subtle physical sensations, clients can bypass cognitive defenses and uncover deeper layers of emotional experience, leading to breakthroughs and transformation.

Gendlin's work was ahead of its time, laying the foundation for modern somatic therapy approaches, which emphasize the connection between the mind and body in healing emotional distress. His contribution to somatic therapy has been highly influential, and I often recommend listening to his audiobook *Focusing* for a deeper, meditative experience of this technique (Gendlin, 1978).

https://focusing.org/sixsteps

1. Clearing a Space
   A. Begin by finding a quiet place and focusing inward.
      • Sit comfortably and allow yourself to relax.
      • Close your eyes and take several deep breaths, noticing how the breath enters and exits your body.
      • Become consciously aware of your breathing, focusing on the sensation of the air filling your lungs and then being released.

   B. Bring attention to your stomach or chest.
      • Ask yourself, "How is my life going? What is the main thing for me right now?"
      • Allow answers to come slowly from within your body, not from your mind.
      • When a concern arises, acknowledge it without going inside it. Stand back and say, "Yes, that's there. I can feel that."

C. Imagine placing each concern in a basket beside you.
- Visualize a basket next to you. As each issue or sensation arises, mentally place it into the basket.
- Continue this process until you feel that every issue, problem, worry, or sensation connected to a situation is in the basket.
- Remember, you are not getting rid of these issues; you are simply moving them from your body at this moment.

D. Identify any background feelings.
- Notice if there is an underlying feeling that is always present, like anxiety, sadness, or a need to keep busy.
- Imagine pulling this feeling down and placing it into the basket as well. This step helps to clear a space for deeper work.

E. Get a bodily sense of the basket's contents.
- Imagine picking up the basket and feeling its weight.
- Put the basket down, allowing yourself to sense its heaviness and how it feels to have these concerns outside of yourself.
- Place the basket away from you—a few feet away, outside a door, or even miles away. Notice any sensations in your body as you do this.

2. Felt Sense
   Choose one problem from the basket to focus on.
- Without going inside it, bring this issue forward and feel it as a whole.
- Pay attention to where you usually feel this problem in your body.
- Observe the overall feeling that comes with this issue, maintaining a distance from it.

3. Handle
   Identify the quality of this unclear felt sense.

- Allow a word, phrase, or image to emerge that captures the essence of the felt sense.
- It might be a quality word like tight, sticky, scary, or an image that represents the feeling.

4. Resonating

   Go back and forth between the felt sense and the word or image.

   - Check how they resonate with each other.
   - Feel for a bodily signal indicating a fit. Let the felt sense and the word or image adjust until they capture the quality just right.

5. Asking:

   Ask what it is about this problem that gives it this quality.

   - Sense the quality again in your body, freshly and vividly.
   - Ask yourself, "What makes the whole problem so?" or "What is in this sense?"
   - If you receive a quick answer without a shift in the felt sense, let it go. Return to the felt sense and ask again until a shift occurs.

6. Receiving

   Welcome whatever comes with a shift.

   - Stay with it for a while, even if it's only a slight release.
   - This is just one shift; there will be others. Continue to stay with the process, allowing time for more awareness and understanding.

By following these detailed steps, you can achieve a deeper understanding and resolution of your issues through bodily awareness and intuitive insight. As Gendlin himself shares,

> If during these instructions somewhere you have spent a little while sensing and touching an unclear holistic body sense of this problem, then you have focused. It doesn't matter whether the

body-shift came or not. It comes on its own. We don't control that.

(1978)

Journaling and Reflections

It's important for you to write down the experience you had during your focusing meditation. By writing out your experience, you will better reflect on the deeper meanings it holds for you. Another powerful way to enhance the healing from this meditation is to draw what you felt or saw. This process helps you take what is inside and externalize it, which creates distance from the parts of yourself that are impacting you. It also offers a greater perspective on the issues that may be preventing you from living your life to the fullest.

Journal about what it was like for you to experience the felt sense of the problem that emerged during your focusing meditation. What insights came to you, and how can you now apply these insights as you move forward?

Dreamwork

Check-in

How has your dream journal been supporting you so far? Have you noticed any shifts in your ability to remember your dreams? As you progress through the fourth module, you may find that your dream recall has intensified (Hill, 2017). This module emphasizes developing a deeper connection to your experiences, and this connection might manifest in how your dreams change and evolve.

Dreams are another form of altered consciousness, and like meditation or Psychedelics, they provide insight into the subconscious (Thompson, 2020). As you continue journaling, take time to reflect on any unusual or significant dreams. Revisit your dream journal and recount anything that feels particularly noteworthy or out of the ordinary.

At times, you may notice that parts of your dreams seem disconnected from the larger narrative. This could be the spirit or energy of the medicine revealing itself, as it often emerges in subtle and symbolic ways (Grof, 2000). By meditating on these disconnected fragments, you might uncover further intuitive messages. Does anything rise to the surface when you focus on these elements?

Using the guidance on page 33, write down any dreams that stand out. Next, circle words that feel significant to you. Even simple words—like "door" or specific colors—may hold symbolic meaning in this reflective process (Jung, 1969a). Pay attention to any bodily sensations or emotional responses as you review these words. Reflect on the themes that emerge, as these might provide clues about your subconscious.

To deepen your connection to the experience or the medicine's energy, ask it to manifest in your dreams before you fall asleep. Keep your journal or recording device close to capture every detail when you wake, including how you feel emotionally. You might also notice moments of déjà vu throughout the day (Dossey, 2001). You don't need immediate answers—just become aware. This practice is a gradual retraining of the brain to develop deeper awareness (Siegel, 2012). By continuing this process of journaling and reflection, you will likely observe shifts in your relationship with your dreams and experience new forms of guidance.

Continuing Your 40-Day Practice

Notice if any changes have occurred as a result of your new routine. As you proceed through this journey of integration, connecting inward will continue to support your growth and expansion. It will also help as you navigate more challenging areas of healing. Even if you haven't begun yet, starting with just one minute a day can make a meaningful shift in your life. In this fast-paced world, we are often expected to give and provide for others. The time you spend in quiet reflection and meditation is time just for you. Whatever method works best for you is perfect. And if you miss a day, don't worry. Simply return to your practice as soon as you remember.

If you've already started, take a moment to reflect: How are you feeling? How are you reacting to others? How has your mood been? Keep track of the changes you notice, both big and small, in your journal. This ongoing reflection will be an essential resource as you continue moving forward in this program.

If you'd like a reminder, you can refer back to page 134 for the instructions for the recommended 40-day practice meditation: **Meditation for an Open Heart**.

Summary: Connecting to the Spirit of the Experience

In this module, we explored the significance of connecting with the spirit of your psychedelic experience, whether it be through plant medicines, synthetic Psychedelics, or other methods of achieving non-ordinary states of consciousness (NOSC). This connection can provide lasting support and resources for integration.

Key Support Elements for Your Journey:

1. **Working Transpersonally:**

    Connecting with a source of energy outside of ourselves (whether through a traditional religious concept of God, or a personal esoteric concept of Nature, Spirit, Source Energy, or other spiritual entities), can provide significant support and nurture your healing journey. This can be specifically relevant to a psychedelic or NOSC as we often experience a connection to something greater than ourselves. Once ingested, the medicine or experience can be seen as a resource that lives within.

    This module discusses how the energy of a non-ordinary state of consciousness can linger long after the experience and ways we can use that energy to support us in our process of moving forward. By tapping into the insights and energy of these experiences, and solidifying them in the body as visceral memories, they can become valuable resources. Whether one believes these experiences originate from a higher power or within oneself, the idea is to access and utilize these memories for ongoing support.

2. **Art Directive—Taking an Inventory of Your Life:**

    You were invited to create a timeline that reflects your past, present, and future using collage images, drawings, and other materials. This exercise is designed to help you explore pivotal moments in your life that you may now want to work towards healing. Additionally, it provides an opportunity to reflect on how your mystical or NOSC experiences may have influenced these moments.

3. **Spiritual Aspects of the Psychedelic Journey:**
    The various profound insights gained from psychedelic experiences, such as a deeper sense of belonging, purpose, and meaning are highlighted here. These experiences can lead to a renewed spirituality, enhanced empathy, and a greater appreciation for life. They also encourage the integration of the Shadow Self and help individuals cope with mortality, accessing the collective unconscious.

4. **Stanislav Grof's Contributions:**
    This module references Stanislav Grof's work, emphasizing the importance of acknowledging transpersonal experiences in therapy. Grof's concept of the "Inner Healer" suggests that patients can access their own deep-seated healing abilities through Psychedelics, guided by a supportive environment.

5. **Meditation: Six Steps of Focusing:**
    This meditation technique helps you get to the root of a problem by identifying inner bodily sensations. Following the detailed steps can lead to a deeper understanding and resolution of issues through bodily awareness and intuitive insight.

6. **Dreamwork:**
    Reflect on your dreams by using art and journaling to explore their meanings. Developing a relationship with your dream state can enhance your ability to remember and integrate these experiences, deepening your awareness and guidance.

In summary, this module provides a comprehensive guide to connecting with the spirit of your psychedelic experience and integrating its insights into your daily life. It emphasizes the importance of maintaining this connection through art, meditation, and reflective practices to support ongoing healing and transformation. By recognizing and nurturing these connections, you foster resilience and sustain your healing journey.

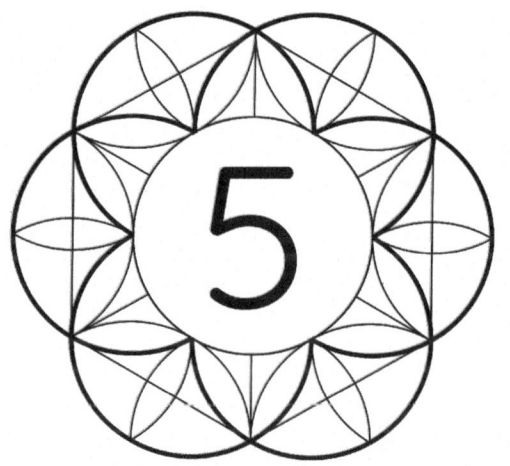

MODULE 5
FALLING IN LOVE WITH SELF

Embracing All Parts of Self as Divine Perfection

Loving yourself can be a profound and challenging journey. After experiencing a Non-ordinary State of Consciousness (NOSC), such as through meditation, breathwork, or psychedelic experiences, you may connect with a deep sense of unconditional love for yourself and others (Grof, 2000). These altered states often bring visions or insights that motivate positive changes. However, there's also the potential to reject parts of yourself—especially the ones that don't align with your desired transformation. It's important to embrace all parts of yourself as aspects of divine perfection, regardless of where you are in your healing journey. Without full self-acceptance, it's difficult to truly love others. When you don't fully love yourself, some parts of you might always feel undeserving of living life fully and joyously (Schwartz, 2020b).

This module focuses on acquiring tools through meditation, reflection, and art-making to help you accept yourself more completely. By accessing self-love, you'll walk your path with greater joy and security in who you are. This will also allow you to open your heart to receive love from others and to share it more freely with those you encounter (Neff, 2011). Connecting and accepting your true Self is a key part of the integration process. As you begin to identify and work with the parts of you that have

 DOI: 10.4324/9781003595762-24

not felt loved, you can offer them the support they need. This can help move you toward deeper and more lasting healing following your NOSC experience (Schwartz and Falconer, 2021).

Psychedelic experiences often allow you to connect with these parts of yourself, offering deeper insights into the areas that need support. Internal Family Systems (IFS), a therapeutic model developed by Schwartz (2020), emphasizes that healing comes through integrating all parts of yourself, including those parts that you might otherwise reject. Throughout this module, you're invited to identify and separate these parts from your core Self or Self-energy so that you can listen to their needs and offer them unconditional love and acceptance (Grof, 2000; Scott, 2015).

One powerful way to access unconditional love is by imagining yourself as a child. According to Scott (2015), we all carry parts of our child-self within us. By acknowledging this inner child, you can begin to offer yourself the kind of pure, unconditional love you might not have received fully. Children embody innocence, curiosity, and wonder; by recognizing and tapping into these qualities within yourself, you can foster self-compassion (Neff, 2011). As you notice what your inner child needs, think about what you, as an adult, can offer. Often, your inner child needs the same thing you might be missing now: to be loved and accepted without condition (Schwartz and Falconer, 2021).

Parts Work: Internal Family Systems (IFS) in Psychedelic Therapy

IFS, developed by Richard Schwartz, Ph.D., conceptualizes the mind as composed of various subpersonalities or "parts," each with its own emotions, beliefs, and agendas. These parts are considered natural elements of the mind but may become extreme or burdensome due to life experiences. In the context of psychedelic therapy, IFS proves especially powerful, as the heightened self-awareness facilitated by Psychedelics allows individuals to access and work with these parts on a deeper level.

By integrating IFS with the three stages of psychedelic therapy—preparation, journey, and integration—and combining it with expressive practices like Art Therapy, clients can achieve profound healing and personal transformation. This model resonates with the expanded states of consciousness induced by Psychedelics, providing an accessible framework to understand and heal the complexities of the mind.

The Essence of Self-Energy

Central to IFS is the concept of "Self" energy. According to Schwartz (2020a), this core aspect of your being is characterized by qualities such as calmness, curiosity, compassion, clarity, confidence, creativity, courage, and connectedness. The Self represents your true essence, distinct from the various parts of your psyche that embody different emotions, beliefs, and coping mechanisms. By accessing and embodying Self-energy, you can navigate life's complexities with far greater balance and cohesion than relying solely on the parts (Schwartz and Falconer, 2021). In psychedelic therapy, connecting with the Self-energy helps individuals navigate challenging experiences with courage and curiosity, facilitating a deeper integration of their psychedelic journeys.

Robert Falconer (2023) elaborates on this by discussing the importance of Self-energy in helping clients not only understand their parts but also to invite spiritual dimensions of healing. He notes that, especially in psychedelic therapy, the "Self" can guide clients through transformative experiences by connecting them with both internal parts and external forces, such as guides or spirit energies, that may appear in psychedelic states.

I often invite individuals I work with to envision Self-energy as the part of them that transcends the physical form, something akin to their Soul or Spirit. Imagine this place within you that embodies inner strength and wisdom, something you can trust completely because it holds the highest intent for your personal journey (Grof, 2000). By developing this relationship, you create a reliable source of guidance—like a friend who supports you through life's challenges. Similar to the guidance you may have received through a psychedelic journey, Self-energy is your birthright and always available (Scott, 2015).

Many of your internal parts, however, may be unaware of the existence of Self-energy. Often, these parts developed during times when Self-energy was inaccessible. As a result, they formed coping strategies to protect the system from external overwhelm. Over time, these protective parts can become distrustful, as they have grown accustomed to managing the system in the absence of Self-energy (Schwartz, 2020b).

These parts—while well-intentioned—often work overtime, guarding against potential threats or emotional distress.

Developing a personal relationship with your Self-energy is crucial. Recognizing where this energy resides within you—perhaps through shapes, colors, or a felt sense—helps strengthen this connection. As you nurture this relationship, Self-energy becomes a reliable inner guide that you can count on when needed. Just like the continued support from an etheric relationship following a psychedelic journey, Self-energy is a fundamental part of your existence and can guide you through life's ups and downs (Schwartz and Falconer, 2021; Scott, 2015).

Accessing Self-Energy

The process of accessing Self-energy involves recognizing and unblending from various parts, particularly those that have taken on protective roles. This can be achieved through a variety of practices:

1. **Mindfulness and Awareness**: Begin with mindfulness practices to increase awareness of internal experiences, recognizing different thoughts, emotions, and bodily sensations (Jones-Callahan, 2016; Schwartz, 2020).

2. **Identifying Parts**: Recognize the parts of yourself that hold various emotions and beliefs, such as a part that feels fear or a part that is critical (Falconer, 2023).

3. **Unblending from Parts**: Gently ask these parts to step back and give space for the Self to emerge. According to Falconer (2023), unblending allows for a clearer perspective where the Self can lead with compassion.

4. **Invoking Self-Qualities**: Consciously bring forward qualities like calmness, compassion, and courage, which are inherent to Self-energy. This practice helps stabilize the mind during both ordinary and altered states of consciousness (Schwartz, 2020a).

5. **Dialoguing with Parts**: Engage in a compassionate dialogue with your parts, acknowledging their fears and needs while offering reassurance from the Self's perspective (Scott, 2022).

6. **Creating Internal Safety**: Cultivate a sense of safety within yourself by assuring parts that Self-energy is capable of leading and

protecting them, a crucial step in IFS and psychedelic integration alike (Falconer, 2023).

7. **Regular Practice**: Just like with any skill, accessing Self-energy improves with consistent practice. Psychedelic therapy offers an accelerated pathway to this, but it's essential to continue engaging with these practices post-journey to ensure sustainable growth (Scott, 2022).

Integrating IFS and Art Therapy into Psychedelic Therapy

1. Preparation: Setting the Stage

   In the preparation phase, you are introduced to the IFS model, where you learn to identify and understand your internal parts or subpersonalities. This is crucial to building a foundation of safety and trust, both with your therapist and within your own internal system (Schwartz, 2020b). You will be introduced to Self-energy, your core essence characterized by calmness, compassion, and curiosity (Falconer, 2023).

   - **Accessing Self Energy**: Through mindfulness practices and guided meditations, you will cultivate an awareness of Self-energy. You'll learn to recognize the different parts within you and approach them with curiosity and empathy. Some of these parts may include your exiles, the wounded or vulnerable parts, or protectors, the parts that keep you safe from emotional harm.

   - **Art Therapy Integration**: Art Therapy is essential at this stage, helping you visualize and externalize your parts. By creating drawings or sculptures of your parts, you can express these aspects in a way that brings deeper understanding and clarity (Scott, 2022). This artistic exploration is important in helping you connect with your Self-energy and understand how your internal system operates (Wallace, 2024).

2. Journey: The Psychedelic Experience

   During the psychedelic experience, altered states of consciousness help you access your internal parts and Self-energy on a much deeper level. Psychedelics break down psychological defenses, allowing for more profound self-awareness (Grof, 2008a).

- **Deep Access to Parts**: The heightened awareness that Psychedelics offer allows you to connect more deeply with your exiles and protectors. These suppressed parts of the psyche often come to the surface, providing an opportunity for healing. Your therapist will support you as you witness these parts without judgment (Schwartz, 2020b). This state of enhanced mental awareness gives you space to explore your inner world and transform your emotional landscape.

- **Art Therapy Integration**: If possible, art-making during or immediately after your psychedelic journey can serve as an outlet for your internal experiences. Creating mandalas or abstract art allows you to process and ground your psychedelic journey through artistic expression (Scott, 2022). Even if making art during the journey is not possible, you can prepare by creating a resource image before the session. This artwork can serve as a guide, reminding you of the Self-energy you carry during the experience.

3. Integration: Bringing It All Together

   The integration phase allows you to process and embed the insights from your psychedelic journey into your everyday life. This is where lasting healing and transformation truly take hold.

   - **Unburdening Exiles**: In the integration phase, you will work to release the burdens carried by your exiles. The connection to Self-energy you develop during the journey allows you to offer compassionate witnessing and validation to these parts, promoting deep healing.

   - **Art Therapy Integration**: Art Therapy becomes a powerful tool for integration. Creating reflective pieces that symbolize your journey from pain to peace allows you to solidify the therapeutic gains (Wallace, 2024). You might create a series of paintings that represent the transformation you've experienced, fostering continued self-reflection and growth (Scott, 2022).

Use the various art directives from this book to expand your awareness of different parts and deepen your understanding of the entire psychedelic journey.

Understanding the Roles of Parts

Proactive Protectors: The Managers

Managers are parts responsible for overseeing daily functions, ensuring you maintain social norms and fulfill responsibilities (Schwartz, 2020a). These parts often emerge early in life, particularly in those who adopted adult roles prematurely, such as parentified children (Scott, 2022). Their main task is to prevent vulnerable exiles from surfacing, using strategies like people-pleasing or avoiding emotional triggers. While their aim is to keep you safe from distress, managers can become rigid and neglect their own needs, creating an imbalance in the internal system.

Reactive Protectors: The Firefighters

Firefighters step in when exiles are triggered, working to quickly distract you from emotional pain by engaging in impulsive behaviors like substance use, overeating, or dissociation (Schwartz, 2020b). These parts prioritize immediate relief, often in conflict with the managers' concern for long-term stability. Firefighters' tactics provide short-term distraction but may create more chronic issues if the exiles' needs remain unaddressed (Falconer, 2023).

Exiles

Exiles carry the emotional weight of past trauma and distress. Often developed in childhood, these parts hold burdens of negative emotions such as guilt, shame, or fear (Schwartz, 2020a). Although pushed aside by protectors to prevent overwhelming the system, exiles influence behaviors and interpretations of situations, often manifesting as physical sensations of heaviness or emotional numbness. Their ultimate desire is to release these painful emotions through a process called "unburdening", which involves compassionate witnessing and integration of positive qualities, allowing for healing and integration within the system (Scott, 2022).

Unburdening Exiles: A Path to Healing

Unburdening exiles is a cornerstone of the IFS model and is crucial for creating a more balanced, harmonious internal system (Falconer, 2023). It allows exiles to release the emotional pain they've carried for years, fostering deeper emotional freedom and healing.

Steps in the Unburdening Process:

1. **Identifying and Accessing Exiles**: Begin by recognizing and approaching exiles with compassion, ensuring a safe space for them to emerge.
2. **Building Trust**: Communicate with the exiles, assuring them that they are safe and will not be abandoned (Schwartz, 2020b).
3. **Witnessing the Pain**: Listen empathetically to the exile's story, validating their emotions while remaining grounded.
4. **Releasing the Burdens**: Use techniques such as visualization or dialogue to help the exile symbolically release their emotional burdens (Scott, 2022).
5. **Integration and Healing**: After the unburdening, reintegrate the exile into your internal system in a healthier, more balanced form.

The Benefits of Unburdening Exiles:

- **Emotional Relief**: Letting go of burdens reduces negative emotions, leading to increased peace and freedom.
- **Improved Relationships**: Healing exiles enhances relationships by reducing reactive behaviors rooted in trauma (Falconer, 2023).
- **Enhanced Self-Awareness**: Unburdening deepens your understanding of your inner world, promoting self-compassion and acceptance.
- **Increased Resilience**: A lighter emotional load improves your ability to face challenges with clarity and strength (Schwartz, 2020a).

Conclusion

Unburdening exiles through the IFS model offers a transformative path to emotional healing and inner harmony, especially when integrated within the stages of psychedelic therapy. By compassionately addressing and releasing the pain carried by these parts, you can experience profound emotional balance, greater self-awareness, and overall well-being (Schwartz, 2020b; Scott, 2022). Art Therapy, integrated into this modality enhances this unburdening process by providing creative and tangible means to explore, express and externalize internal experiences (Wallace, 2024). Together, the use of IFS, Art Therapy, and psychedelic experiences creates a powerful opportunity to reclaim wholeness and live with deeper fulfillment and emotional freedom. As Richard Schwartz reminds us, "Within you is a family of selves, each with its own story. Embrace them all with love and curiosity."

Art Directive: Mandalas as a Reflection of Self

Materials Needed:

- Art materials such as paints, pastels, crayons, colored pencils, markers, or any drawing materials of your choice.
- A medium to heavyweight piece of paper cut in the shape of a perfect circle, anywhere from 5" to 12" in diameter.

Instructions:

- Mandalas can assist with meditation and enhance personal awareness (Fincher, 2010).
- Mandalas, a Sanskrit word for "circle," are symbols that have been used by various cultures, including Hinduism and Buddhism, to represent the universe and aid in meditation (Jung, 1973). You can work with mandalas to deepen your meditation practice or simply decorate them with symbols that hold personal significance (Kellogg, 1992). These symbols can serve as reminders throughout your living space.
- The circle, as a symbol, represents wholeness and oneness across many cultures. It embodies the indivisible fulfillment of the universe, symbolizing unity and total completeness (Jung, 1964).
- The essence of the circle transcends linear thinking, encompassing holistic perspectives, feelings, and intuitions. Like the circle, these

perspectives have a greater wisdom beyond the finite elements contained within them. The circle is a profound symbol; other geometries and symbols reflect different aspects of its absolute perfection (Husum, 2023).

- With your circular piece of paper in front of you, begin drawing within your mandala. You can create repeating patterns or simply draw whatever symbols, shapes, or colors resonate with you (Kellogg, 1992). This mandala is your personal "Representation of Self," and there are no wrong ways to create it. Carl Jung first described this method used with himself and patients outlined in "The Red Book", (Jung, 2009).
- Continue creating until you feel a sense of completion.

Now That You've Finished Your Mandala Art Activity:

- Once you've finished your mandala, take a moment to observe the colors you used. Reflect on the predominant colors and those used sparingly.
- Observe the images and shapes you've drawn—pay attention to any contrasts, hard or soft lines, and jagged or smooth edges.
- Write down your feelings and any memories or associations that arise when you reflect on the colors, shapes, and designs in your mandala. Connections between your mandala and the emotions or sensations you experienced while creating it may emerge (Kornfield, 2009).
- Remember, this process is deeply personal and introspective. Your mandala is a symbol of who you were at the moment of its creation, reflecting your inner landscape (Jung, 1973).

Journaling and Reflections:

- Use your journal to reflect on how the creation process felt for you. If you feel comfortable, consider sharing your thoughts with your therapist or a trusted friend (Fincher, 2010).
- Notice any emotions that surface as you revisit the colors and shapes of your mandala. Do they bring up any memories or associations (Kellogg, et al.,1977)?

- Ask yourself if the shapes or colors bring you back to a different time or place.
- Sit with these feelings as they arise, knowing you are supported. You can always tap into your resource image for protection and guidance. Trust your inner wisdom, recognizing that you and your experiences have meaning and purpose.

Art Directive: Understanding and Accepting Self

Materials Needed:

- Mirror
- Marker, pencil, crayon, chalk pastel, etc. (Choose two to begin with)
- 2 large pieces of medium-weight paper

Self-Portrait with Non-Dominant Hand

Engaging in a self-portrait using your non-dominant hand is a powerful art directive for viewing yourself from a new perspective and embracing both your strengths and flaws. This directive is sometimes referred to as a *"Blind Contour Drawing"*, exemplified in the works of Elizabeth Layton (1984). By using the non-dominant hand, you invite a level of vulnerability that can promote self-compassion and encourage deeper acceptance of your true self (Layton, 1984). This practice bypasses the familiar thinking mind, allowing the brain to navigate from unfamiliar territory, helping to access a range of feelings, insights, and self-acceptance that may not have been previously available.

This method of using art as a form of self-reflection and emotional processing is supported by therapeutic approaches like Gestalt Art Therapy, which emphasizes the here-and-now experience and how it is expressed through creativity (Carpendale, 2023). Additionally, using self-portraits as a tool in Art Therapy, as Moon (2002c) describes, allows for deeper self-exploration and personal insight. Drawing with the non-dominant hand can access subconscious feelings, bypassing the usual cognitive defenses (Cameron, 1992), making it an effective practice for emotional and psychological healing.

By using the non-dominant hand, you're inviting new layers of understanding about yourself, which can deepen your connection to self-acceptance and compassion.

Part A: Drawing with Non-Dominant Hand

1. Using your non-dominant hand and either a marker, pencil, chalk pastel, or any material and color you like.
2. While looking in the mirror, take one material and, **without lifting your hand**, begin drawing your face on the paper. This again, is done with the non-dominant hand.
3. Be careful if judgments come up and acknowledge that this exercise is not about creating the most beautiful drawing. It is about expressing with a side of you that doesn't always have the opportunity to express itself, your non-dominant side.
4. Notice any feelings or sensations that come up in your body and just allow these to pass, feeling a sense of love and acceptance with each sensation.
5. When finished, take a moment to look at your drawing as if a child you loved drew this for you, with all of their heart.

Part B: Drawing with Dominant Hand

1. Using another color and even a different medium if this feels right, look into your mirror, and now create a self-portrait of what you see with your dominant hand, careful not to lift your writing device from the paper, creating this image with one continuous line.
2. Again, notice any sensations that arise in the body, paying attention to them with loving acceptance. Stay connected to your breath and the process you are experiencing in the moment.
3. Once finished with your drawing, stand back from both of them and notice the differences. Notice what you would like to change or alter or areas you really like and would like to keep as they are. What stands out for you? What messages arise? Notice the beautiful aspects of your creation, of you, and write these down.

Part C: Alter and Reflect

1. With both portraits in front of you, now use any materials or colors that feel right and alter your drawings in whatever way resonates with you. Add to or change elements, embellish certain parts, or leave others as they are.

2. Reflect on how you are able to make changes and embrace what you want to keep. Allow yourself to notice the freedom to evolve your artwork as you see fit.

3. Once you feel your artwork is complete, sit quietly with both portraits. Go inward and observe the emotions that surface. Breathe into these feelings and allow them to release and flow through you.

4. Use your journal to write any reflections that come to mind. Consider what messages you've received from your art or the process itself. These could be insights into how you see yourself or how you feel about the act of creation.

Meditation for Greater Self-Love

This powerful meditation practice is designed to unlock the heart, cultivate a positive self-relationship, and prepare oneself to receive and give love abundantly.

Part 1

This initial phase focuses on a process of self-blessing designed to align and purify the body's magnetic field, or aura. If you're holding onto unresolved anger, this meditation may help to release it, which can sometimes cause discomfort as you move through the practice. Stay connected to your breath and grounded to the earth, allowing yourself to move through these sensations. However, always listen to your body—if you experience sharp pain, stop immediately. You might also notice a change in taste in your mouth, which is completely normal. Keep breathing deeply and allow the inner workings of this meditation to take hold.

Posture:

- Sit in Easy Pose (cross-legged on the floor) with a straight spine, or in a chair with feet on the ground.
- Hold your right palm six to nine inches above the top center of your head, facing down as if blessing you. This self-blessing is intended to strengthen and balance your auric energy.
- The left elbow is bent with the upper arm near the rib cage. The forearm and hand point up with the left palm facing forward as if giving a pledge, with the intent of blessing the world around you.

Eyes:

- With closed eyes, focus your gaze at the tip of the chin, the lunar center.

Breath:

- Breathe with full extended slow breaths while imagining a feeling of deep affection for self with each inhale and exhale.
- As you breathe, regulate the timing of your breath so there is an even amount of inhale, suspension of the breath, and exhale. See if you can work towards having one full breath per minute: Inhale for 20 seconds, hold for 20 seconds, exhale for 20 seconds.

Time:

- Continue for 11 minutes.
- Then inhale fully and move slowly and directly into position for Exercise 2.

Part 2

The second phase of this meditation concentrates on the region encompassing the neck and navel. Working on the Heart center, it allows this region to strengthen and open to an expanded love of self.

Posture:

- Stretch your arms out in front of you, parallel to the ground, with your palms facing down. Feel yourself stretching to your maximum.

Eyes:

- The eyes are closed and remain focused on the lunar center in the center of the chin.
- Breath:
- The breath is full, slow, and rhythmic.

Time:

- Continue for 3 minutes. Then inhale deeply and move slowly and directly into position for the third phase of this meditation.

Part 3

Posture:

- Reach the arms straight up above the head with the palms facing forward, fingertips together, extended upward. Keep the elbows straight.

Eyes:

- The eyes are closed and focused on the lunar center: the tip of the chin.
- Breath:
- The breath continues with full, slow, and rhythmic breaths.

Time:

- Continue for 3 minutes.

To Finish

- Take a full inhale and suspend the breath as you stretch your arms upward to your maximum (try to stretch so much that your buttocks are lifted) while tightening all the muscles of your body. With closed eyes, feel your gaze shift to the top of your head. Hold the breath as you stretch. Exhale and release the stretch. Repeat with this full inhale and stretch while tensing all muscles, two more times.

By fully engaging in each phase of this meditation intended to cultivate a love of self, you are supported in opening your heart to create a sense of compassion for yourself that is your birthright. Notice the shifts in your life as you open your heart and become more open to receiving love in all of its forms.

Journaling and Reflections

As you continue to reflect on the parts within yourself that may have surfaced throughout this module, particularly with a focus on loving yourself, consider which parts may want to speak. Externalizing your thoughts and emotions—whether through art materials or journaling—can deepen your understanding and allow for new insights to emerge.

Step 1: Grounding and Connecting with Self Energy

Start by sitting quietly after a brief meditation or grounding exercise. This practice is meant to help you connect to your *Self-energy*—a central concept in IFS therapy, which as mentioned, refers to your core essence that embodies qualities like calmness, curiosity, and compassion (Schwartz, 2020a). Tune in to where this energy resides in your body and notice its qualities: Is there a color, shape, or texture that represents your Self energy? Allow your breath to flow into this space, enhancing the connection.

Step 2: Inviting Other Parts to Speak

Once you feel connected to your Self energy, invite any other parts that may want to come forward. It is important to remain curious and compassionate toward these parts, allowing them to express what they want to share. You can use different colored pens for each part, distinguishing their voices from that of your Self energy. This creates an opportunity for each part to be acknowledged and heard.

- **Ask your parts** what roles they play within your system. Remember, as Richard Schwartz emphasizes in IFS, "there are no bad parts" (Schwartz, 2020b). Each part has a protective role, even if its methods may seem challenging.
- **Thank your parts** for their efforts and observe their reactions. Offering gratitude to these parts can foster a sense of trust and ease.
- **Ask them when they were born.** Often, parts emerge as coping mechanisms during childhood, when there was no access to Self-energy. Understanding their origin can provide context and clarity.
- **Ask how old they think you are now.** If their perception of your age differs from your current reality, update them. This can help recalibrate their understanding and alleviate some of their burdens.

Step 3: Offering Self Energy

Let your parts know that you now have access to your Self-energy, which is here to care for them. Many parts develop when Self-energy was unavailable, so it can take time for them to trust that it is present now (Schwartz, 2020a; Falconer, 2023). Be patient as they adjust, and if they are open to it, offer them some of your Self-energy to reassure them that they are safe.

Step 4: Shifting Roles

Ask your parts if there is something they would rather be doing if they were not working so hard in your system to support it and protect you. Invite them to do this, letting them know that you now have Self-energy and can do the job they have been so tirelessly doing for so long. Many parts, particularly those formed in response to trauma, may feel overworked and burdened (Scott, 2021). Allow them the freedom to step aside, letting Self-energy take on the job they have been doing for so long. Be clear that you are not trying to get rid of them, they have been working hard and play an important role in your system but it is ok for them to soften and step aside. Self-energy is now here to keep your system balanced and supported.

Conclusion: Cultivating Relationships with Your Parts

As you develop relationships with your parts, they no longer feel so enmeshed within your system and you are able to develop greater control for when they may take over. When fully activated, parts can morph into personality traits that feel like the whole self, when in reality, they are just aspects of Self wanting to help. This process of dialoguing with your parts, and fostering trust, allows them to function as helpful "parts" rather than defining your entire identity.

Continuing Your 40-Day Practice

You've come halfway through this book and although it is your choice to dive into a dedicated practice at any point, if you have followed this up until now, I imagine you are noticing some profound shifts. If you have not yet begun, give it a try, even if it's just one minute a day. Do something in a quiet state of meditation and reflection that will support you. See this as a gift you give to yourself on your path of integration and ultimately a life filled with abundant joy. This does not need to be an activity that you feel pressure to do, but rather something that gives more to you than the time it takes.

If you have already begun, continue to track any shifts or changes in the way you are in the world. Have your interactions with others or yourself changed? Stay open, with curiosity about how quiet reflection and meditation are rerouting the neuropathways in your brain. How are you feeling? How are you reacting to others? How has your mood been? Keep notice of the changes that are beginning and continuing to form. This will be of great support as we move through the protocols offered in this book.

If you'd like, you can return back to page 134 and onward for the instructions for the recommended 40-day practice meditation: Meditation for an Open Heart.

Summary: Falling in Love with Self

Module Five delves into the profound journey of achieving true self-love. After experiencing non-ordinary states of consciousness (NOSC), many people connect to a sense of unconditional love for themselves and others. These experiences often reveal parts of ourselves that we feel motivated to change. However, it's essential to accept all parts of ourselves as divine perfection, regardless of our stage of healing. Without this acceptance, it is challenging to fully love others and embrace a life filled with joy. This chapter deepens the integration process by acknowledging and accepting the parts of Self we may not always understand or hear.

Key Support Elements for Your Journey:

1. **Embracing All Parts of Self as Divine Perfection:**
   This module introduces the concept of viewing all parts of the Self as expressions of divine perfection. It explores the challenges and rewards of cultivating true self-love, especially following a Non-Ordinary State of Consciousness (NOSC) experience. It emphasizes that accepting all aspects of oneself is key to both personal healing and the ability to fully love others, ultimately leading to a more fulfilling life.

2. **Parts Work: IFS in Psychedelic Therapy:**
   This chapter delves into the IFS therapy model, which views the mind as composed of various subpersonalities or "parts." It explores how IFS can be integrated with psychedelic therapy to facilitate profound healing. In particular, aspects within this therapy covered are:
   • Accessing Self-Energy
   • Integrating IFS and Art Therapy
   • Understanding the Roles of Parts
   • Unburdening Exiles

3. **Art Directive: Mandalas as a Reflection of Self:**
   This module introduces the use of mandalas as an art directive for self-reflection and exploration. Drawing from somatic approaches, you are invited to create a mandala as a meditative practice that fosters personal awareness. The process of mandala creation serves as a visual and creative pathway to connect with the inner Self, promoting a deeper sense of unity, balance, and completeness (Jung, 2009).

4. **Art Directive: Understanding and Accepting Self:**
   This art directive focuses on self-portraiture as a method for understanding and accepting oneself. It includes exercises that involve drawing oneself using both the non-dominant and dominant hands, encouraging readers to explore their perceptions of self and to embrace both their strengths and flaws with compassion and acceptance (Layton, 1984).

5. **Meditation for Loving Self:**
   A powerful meditation practice designed to unlock the heart, cultivate a positive self-relationship, and prepare oneself to give and receive love abundantly. The meditation is broken down into several phases, each aimed at aligning and purifying the body's magnetic field, opening the heart center, and fostering a deeper connection to Self-energy.

6. **Journaling and Reflections:**
   As we continue through the integration process, you are encouraged to engage in journaling as a means of reflecting on the insights gained throughout the module. The process of moving thoughts and feelings from within to the outside—whether through writing or art—facilitates deeper understanding and allows new awareness to emerge. The chapter provides prompts and guidance for reflective journaling to enhance the journey towards self-love.

7. **Continuing Your 40-Day Practice:**
   You are encouraged to continue and reflect on what changes are happening for you with your 40-day meditation and reflection practice, as introduced earlier in the program. Emphasizing the importance of consistency in this practice, as you notice any profound shifts happening in how you interact with yourself and others.

By fully engaging in the practices and directives presented in this module, individuals are supported in opening their hearts to create a sense of compassion for themselves, fostering a deeper connection to self and others.

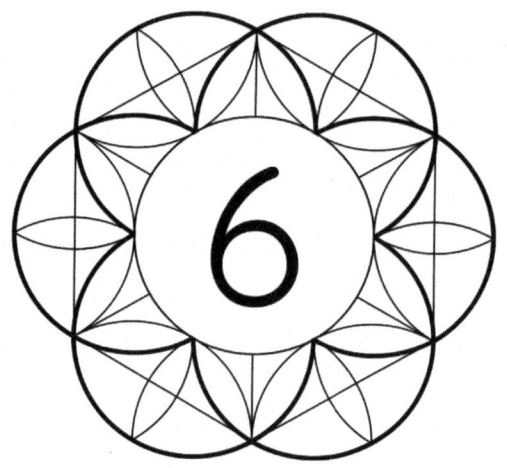

Module 6
Understanding Our Attachment Styles

In this module, we are moving deeply into the process of Integration. For many of the clients I see, the theme of healing early attachment patterning wounds becomes central to creating inner awareness and lasting healing, which the medicine opens one to. The psychological frameworks of attachment theory and inner child healing can significantly enrich the process of psychedelic therapy as we dive into the areas within life that may be causing disruptions for us.

Notice what comes up for you as you read through and experience this module and the art directives shared. How might your life change or be supported as you explore your own inner healing? The medicine opens that window, and now we do the deeper work into the Integration process.

Understanding Attachment Styles

Attachment styles have become a key focus in understanding how we form relationships, particularly in the realm of psychotherapy and personal development. The way we connect with others—and maintain those connections—is essential to the human experience. These patterns of attachment are largely influenced by the first seven years of life, during which caregivers play a central role in shaping how we perceive love, safety, and connection (Proulx, 2017). In this module, we will explore different attachment styles and examine how they impact adult relationships.

DOI: 10.4324/9781003595762-25   193

Attachment theory, originally developed by John Bowlby, has evolved significantly over time and remains essential for understanding relationship dynamics. Psychedelic therapy can deepen this understanding by providing access to early relational traumas and attachment wounds (Woolley, 2017). Through revisiting past experiences in altered states and during the integration process, individuals are able to reprocess attachment issues and potentially rewire their attachment patterns (Levine and Frederick, 1997). The awareness and insights gained from psychedelic journeys can help individuals develop more secure attachment behaviors, form healthier relationships, and improve emotional regulation.

Notice which patterns resonate with you as you read through this chapter. By recognizing patterns that are playing out subconsciously in life, there is an opportunity to move beyond and through them.

Key Attachment Styles Generally, people fall into three main attachment styles, with a fourth, less common style:

1. **Anxious**
2. **Avoidant**
3. **Secure**
4. **Disorganized (Anxious-Avoidant)**

In the section that follows this, we will look closer at how these attachment styles are created and ways of giving ourselves, as adults, the nurturing needed to move into a Secure Attachment style. Feeling secure in the way we connect with others will help to bring more harmonious and balanced relationships and friendships into our lives.

We may have different patterns with different people. The important thing is to know ourselves well enough to spot when we are unconsciously acting from dysfunctional conditioned patterning. By recognizing how we relate to others in the world and taking responsibility for our actions, we are able to show up in a more authentic and secure way.

Anxious or Preoccupied Attachment Style

- Characterized by a persistent fear of rejection and abandonment, individuals with an anxious attachment style may become preoccupied with their relationships, seeking constant reassurance (Mikulincer and Shaver, 2007). The root of this insecurity often lies in unresolved childhood experiences where caregivers may have been inconsistently available or emotionally unpredictable.

- Feelings of fear, hurt, anger, and rejection from unresolved past issues from one's family of origin begin to intrude into present perceptions of one's relationship with a core belief that "it will happen again."
- This attachment style often results in heightened emotional reactivity and struggles with personal boundaries, leading to a dynamic where one constantly seeks validation from a partner.
- There can be a desire to "merge" with the other that can, in turn, scare a partner away.
- Individuals with anxious attachment may have difficulty seeing their own role in conflicts, placing blame on others while feeling highly sensitive to their partner's moods and behaviors.
- Becoming highly emotional, argumentative, combative, angry, and controlling with poor personal boundaries.
- One's moods become unpredictable, with a predisposition for connecting through conflict or "stirring the pot" to get a reaction.
- Taking a partner's behavior too personally and becoming overly sensitive to another's moods and actions.
- Continuously blaming others and unaware of one's own responsibility in issues that arise in the relationship. Communication is not collaborative but one-sided and rigid.
- Inconsistent attunement with one's own children, who are likely to be anxiously attached.

Avoidant, Dismissive, or Ambivalent Attachment Style

- People with an avoidant attachment style tend to avoid emotional closeness, fearing it will lead to a loss of independence. They may push partners away, often finding faults in the other, as a way of maintaining emotional distance and self-reliance (Levine and Heller, 2010).

- Avoidant individuals may rely on intellectual communication rather than emotional expression, often suppressing or avoiding feelings in both relationships and conflicts (Schore, 2012).
- One may avoid conflict or healthy communication but then explode with anger, further justifying the blockage in connection.
- Counter-dependence in which a person refuses to depend on the other and establishes rigid boundaries, never seeking help and not allowing their partner to lean on them.
- In a crisis, a person with this attachment style remains non-emotional, taking charge and handling situations well without emotion.
- This style of attachment is often characterized by a preference for being alone, staying cool, controlled, stoic, and compulsively self-sufficient with a narrow emotional range.
- As a parent, emotionally unavailable, disengaged, and detached. Children of parents with this attachment style are likely to also develop an avoidant attachment style.
- This attachment pattern often emerges in individuals whose caregivers were emotionally unavailable or dismissive, leading them to internalize the belief that vulnerability is dangerous.

Secure Attachment Style

- Securely attached individuals are comfortable with intimacy and independence, forming balanced, emotionally supportive relationships (Siegel, 2012). They are able to communicate openly and honestly with their partners and are attuned to their emotional needs.
- This attachment style usually develops when a caregiver provides consistent emotional support and is responsive to a child's needs.
- People with secure attachment styles tend to feel emotionally balanced and can handle relational challenges without becoming overwhelmed.
- In a secure attachment pattern, one is tolerant of differences, forgiving, trusting, and empathic.
- Communication comes easily, and one is able to express their needs honestly and openly. They are attuned to their partner's needs and respond appropriately while not avoiding conflict.

- The person is available for their partner in times of need and is not afraid to depend on another and be dependable themselves.
- The person is accepting of and doesn't feel rejected or threatened when their partner needs time alone and is okay with being independent of their partner while still feeling close.
- Past relationship issues and hurts have brought insight to a person with a secure attachment style where resolution and forgiveness have been attained.
- One is balanced emotionally and does not become overly upset about relationship issues.
- Children of a securely attached person are also securely attached. This person is attuned to their child's cues and needs and is a sensitive, warm, and caring parent.

Disorganized Attachment Style

- Disorganized attachment, a combination of anxious and avoidant behaviors, often results from experiences of trauma or abuse in early childhood (Liotti, 2004). These individuals may have learned to fear their caregiver, creating conflicting needs for both closeness and distance.
- In relationships, this attachment style often manifests as unpredictable or erratic behavior, where individuals may crave intimacy yet push it away out of fear of being hurt.
- Emotional closeness in a relationship is unbearable, resulting in an inability to regulate emotions with a quickness to become argumentative and full of rage. Past patterns are recreated through abusive and dysfunctional relationships.
- The losses one has experienced from the past have not been mourned or resolved, and one is still very frightened by the memories of prior traumas, which cause emotional upsets.
- One may experience severe depression and symptoms of PTSD (Post-Traumatic Stress Disorder) with dissociative habits to avoid feeling pain. Frightening, traumatic memories are intrusive and easily triggered.

- One's own children may develop a disorganized attachment style as parents with this attachment style have a higher probability of treating their kids the way they too were treated. Parents may quickly become triggered by their children, projecting their own abuses they experienced in childhood.
- People with this style of attachment are often narcissistic with antisocial behavior and a lack of empathy and remorse for others. They can be aggressive and punitive with no regard for rules and may also be prone to substance abuse and even criminality.

Healing Through Awareness and Integration

Our attachment patterns begin in childhood and are passed down from one generation to the next. Children learn how to connect with parents and caregivers, and they, in turn, teach the next generation. Your attachment history plays a crucial role in determining how you relate to your adult relationships and how you relate to your children. However, it is not what happened to you as a child that matters most—it is how you deal with it. The idea that adverse life experiences can empower us to utilize the skills necessary to overcome them has been proven time and time again.

Recognizing one's attachment style is the first step in breaking free from the subconscious patterns that shape our relationships (Proulx, 2017). Psychedelic therapy can offer profound insights into these attachment wounds, helping individuals to reprocess early trauma and develop a more secure attachment style (Carhart-Harris et al., 2018a). By facing these issues in an altered state of consciousness and processing them during integration, individuals can break free from dysfunctional cycles and create more authentic, healthy, and balanced connections with others. Through this process, we can move from insecure attachment patterns toward greater emotional stability and relational harmony.

Somatically Experiencing Life

Somatically experiencing life begins with becoming aware of sensations within *your* body and the messages they carry. This awareness is crucial for health, emotional regulation, and the ability to fully engage with life. However, many of us have learned to ignore or override these internal cues, focusing instead on external validations, like how others see us, our appearance, or material possessions. In an attempt to feel more confident, you may define yourself by thoughts and ideas, giving more importance to what the mind thinks rather than what is felt within. This disconnect from your inner self can leave you feeling empty, searching for a sense of self in external actions or relationships, and preventing you from building trust in *your* Self-energy.

Learning to trust your body's signals and reconnect with your true Self-energy brings stability and balance, allowing you to navigate life's challenges with a sense of control and groundedness. When you tap into this level of awareness, learning to understand and trust the messages from your inner voice becomes a powerful strength. This somatic awareness gives you access to authentic self-experience, which Levine (2010) describes as essential for healing trauma. When you are attuned to your body, you can better manage intense emotions, make informed choices, and live more authentically.

Yet, for some, the body doesn't always feel safe. Traumatic experiences can lead to dissociation—a protective mechanism that causes a detachment from bodily sensations, making it difficult to stay grounded in the present moment (Levine, 2010). This dissociation can prevent you from accessing Self-energy, which is critical for navigating life's complexities with resilience and compassion (Schwartz, 2020a).

In the context of psychedelic therapy, this reconnection with the body can be even more profound. Psychedelics and other Non-Ordinary States of Consciousness can help unlock deep-seated trauma by facilitating a heightened sense of somatic awareness (Carhart-Harris and Friston, 2019). In these altered states, you are often able to reconnect with sensations that were previously blocked or repressed, enabling you to confront and heal trauma. Through these journeys, you learn to titrate—moving back and forth between feelings of safety and discomfort—allowing your body to slowly become a place of safety once again (Levine, 2010).

Psychedelic therapy provides a unique opportunity to bridge this gap. By combining somatic practices with the expansive awareness Psychedelics offer, you can foster a deep reconnection with your inner wisdom and bodily awareness. Instead of looking outward for validation, you begin to trust yourself, building a stronger, more secure sense of self that allows for greater authenticity and emotional resilience.

Recreating Our Primary Scenario

Primary Scenario Arena

A term used in Integrative Body Psychotherapy (IBP), this space looks into your childhood, exploring the patterns in relationships and how you saw yourself and others as you grew up. The blueprints for how you handle intimacy, your well-being, and your views on sexuality were created during this time. Babies pick up their parents' attitudes, moods, desires, and needs through unspoken "parent messages", conveyed not through words but through presence, emotions, and touch. These messages, if received from caring parents boost confidence, self-worth, and the ability to form close relationships. Parents who received these messages naturally pass them on, while those who didn't face more challenges.

The "Good Parent Messages," originated by Jack Lee Rosenberg, Ph.D., and Beverly Kitaen Morse, Ph.D., through their work in IBP, serve as powerful affirmations that nurture and reparent the inner child. These messages are meant to cultivate a secure sense of self by addressing unmet emotional needs from early childhood (Rosenberg et al., 1989). By speaking these messages aloud, you invite healing through self-compassion and reprogramming.

These affirmations are meant to re-establish an internal sense of security, allowing you to internalize the unconditional support that may have been absent during childhood. Each message creates experiences felt in various parts of the body. Learning to recognize and experience these feelings involves tuning into your body, not just relying on your mind. As you say each one aloud, notice any discomfort or resistance. These reactions can indicate areas where the message wasn't often heard but is now needed (Rosenberg et al., 1989). If you didn't hear them as a child, offer these to yourself now. In practicing these affirmations, you begin the process of reparenting your inner child, offering the safety and love necessary for deep emotional healing.

Good Parent Messages[1]

Earliest Childhood Messages:

Speak these messages aloud and notice the different sensations that arise in the body.

- I love you
- I want you
- You are special to me.
- I see you and hear you
- It is not what you do but who you are that I love.
- I love you and give you permission to be different from me.
- I'll take care of you.
- I'll be there for you; I will be there even when you die.
- You don't have to be alone anymore.
- You can trust me.
- You can trust your inner voice.
- Sometimes I will tell you "No," and that's because I love you.
- You don't have to be afraid anymore.
- My love will make you well
- I welcome and cherish your love.

Research on early childhood attachment underscores the significant role of such positive affirmations from caregivers in shaping secure attachment and emotional regulation (Siegel and Hartzell, 2014; Schore, 2019). Messages like these build a foundation for a healthy sense of self, enabling individuals to grow with a secure attachment style and emotional resilience (Bowlby, 1988).

Out In the World Messages:

1. I can set limits, and I am willing to enforce them.
2. If you fall down, I will pick you up.
3. I am proud of you.
4. I have confidence in you, I am sure you will succeed.
5. I give you permission to be the same as I, to be more or less.
6. You are beautiful (or handsome)
7. I give you permission to love and enjoy your erotic sexuality with a partner of your choice and not lose me.

The importance of such affirmations, particularly around setting boundaries and expressing love unconditionally, can impact an individual's emotional development and self-concept (Perry and Szalavitz, 2017). For instance, affirmations around confidence and boundaries are vital for the development of autonomy and self-regulation (Erikson, 1950; Shaver and Mikulincer, 2012).

Reflection and Integration of Messages

Imagine how different your life might be if you had received these affirmations consistently from childhood and were no longer compelled to seek them externally. These messages can profoundly shape your emotional and psychological development, helping you cultivate an internal sense of worth and security (Neff, 2011).

As you read each message aloud, reflect on which ones feel challenging to receive. Did any cause a disconnection, i.e., did you find your mind wandering as you read it aloud? This unconscious reaction is often a sign that a Good Parent Message was one you did not hear often enough or one that would be helpful for you to hear more. These messages, while simple, address deep-rooted needs for safety, love, and connection, which attachment research suggests are critical for well-being (Schore, 2019). You are the parent now of your own inner child, so allow these messages to be felt completely; allow them to sink into your body.

Next Steps

If you'd like to deepen this work, consider writing out the messages that are difficult for you to internalize. Place them on post-it notes in areas you can see regularly as a way to consciously integrate these affirmations into your daily life. This practice echoes the principles of self-compassion and cognitive restructuring, which are often used in therapeutic settings to foster positive self-talk and healing (Neff, 2011; Gilbert, 2014). The work you are doing now will support you in your process of growth and transformation that will stay with you for a lifetime. Celebrate the work you are doing, recognizing the younger parts within you that are feeling more loved and cared for each day. If you need extra support, be sure to reach out to someone you trust. Have faith that the inner strength is within you and burning brighter with each day!

How Do Secure Attachment Patterns Develop?

For a child to develop emotional stability and resilience, both the child and their caregivers must collaborate on three essential tasks:

1. **Form a Bond**: Building a strong emotional bond between a child and their primary caregiver is foundational. This bond provides the child with a sense of security, trust, and love. If this bond isn't formed, the child may develop emotional wounds that lead to anxiety and an ongoing fear of abandonment (Schore, 2003; Bowlby, 1988).

2. **Develop Empathic Attunement**: Parents and children need to understand each other on an emotional level. This attunement allows for a harmonious relationship where the child's emotions are validated, and the child feels seen and heard (Siegel, 2012).

3. **Allow Sufficient Space**: It's equally crucial for parents to provide enough space for their child to develop autonomy. Giving children the freedom to explore and establish their own identity builds confidence and nurtures their curiosity and safety (Schore, 2003).

In healthy relationships, balancing these three components is ongoing. However, when they are not achieved during childhood, the child may carry emotional scars into adulthood, which can shape their attachment style.

The Bond: Abandonment Anxiety

Creating a secure bond with caregivers is vital for children to develop trust in both others and themselves. This bond helps children believe that they are worthy of love and ensures that they will not be abandoned (Bowlby, 1988). Without it, the natural need for connection can become exaggerated, leading to a profound fear of abandonment in adulthood.

This can manifest in intimate relationships as an overwhelming need for reassurance and connection, often resulting in behaviors that strain relationships. The fear of abandonment can become a self-fulfilling prophecy if left unchecked, as these behaviors push partners away, ultimately causing the very abandonment that was feared (Schore, 2003).

Breathing Room: Inundation (Avoidant) Anxiety

Children also need room to explore their individuality. Without the space to make their own decisions, test their abilities, and learn from their mistakes, they may struggle to establish a sense of self. Over-controlling parents, or "helicopter parenting," can make a child feel suffocated and unable to develop autonomy. In these cases, children may grow into adults who feel trapped in relationships, leading to avoidant behaviors (Siegel, 2012).

As adults, those who experience this kind of over-control may sabotage relationships by distancing themselves from their partners or avoiding emotional intimacy altogether. These patterns are a result of childhood inundation, where they were not allowed the freedom to be themselves (Schore, 2003). Any attempts by others to offer closeness or affection might be interpreted as control or manipulation, triggering feelings of entrapment.

Which Character Style Do You Identify With?

Abandonment character styles typically involve clinging within relationships, while avoidant character styles result in pushing others away. When these two anxieties are at odds, attunement—the experience of mutuality, reciprocity, and shared experience—becomes difficult. High levels of abandonment anxiety are temporarily relieved by getting closer to someone, while inundation or avoidant anxiety is eased by creating distance.

Abandonment Anxiety

In relationships, abandonment anxiety can manifest in various unhealthy patterns, such as:

- Acquiescence: *I will do anything; just don't leave me.*
- Eternal Longings: *No matter what, it's never enough.*
- Diffuse Boundaries: *There's no such thing as too close.*
- Clinging: *Constantly orbiting around someone or something.*
- Hyper-Vulnerability: *Acutely aware of emotions and sensations in the body.*

According to attachment theory, these tendencies often arise from inconsistent caregiving in early childhood, where the child may feel unsure about whether their emotional needs will be met (Ainsworth and Bowlby, 1991). Without secure attachment, this can translate into an anxious preoccupation with maintaining closeness in adulthood (Mikulincer and Shaver, 2007).

Inundation Anxiety (Avoidant Patterns)

In contrast, individuals with inundation or avoidant anxiety character styles tend to display traits such as:

- Separate and Removed: *I am what I am.*
- Emotional Detachment: *Cut off from feelings and emotions.*
- Rigid Boundaries: *Rigid and impenetrable emotional barriers.*
- Black-and-White Assumptions: *Viewing the world in stark contrasts.*
- Physical and Emotional Armor: *Maintaining a tough exterior.*

These avoidant traits are rooted in early childhood experiences where caregivers may have been emotionally distant or overwhelmed, leaving the child to fend for themselves emotionally. As a result, the adult develops a defensive strategy, relying on emotional distance as a means of self-preservation (Bowlby, 1988; Mikulincer and Shaver, 2007).

Agency and Codependency

An "agent" in IBP terms refers to someone who feels compelled to meet the needs of others at the expense of their own identity and desires. Over time, this can lead to physical and emotional exhaustion, as well as a diminished sense of self (Rosenberg and Kitaen-Morse, 2004b).

Agency often develops in childhood, particularly in cases where children are forced to take on caregiving roles for their parents. This reversal of roles results in the development of co-dependent traits, where the child believes their survival depends on tending to the emotional needs of the parent (Scott, 2022a). As a result, self-agency— the ability to make decisions and feel a sense of personal control—takes a back seat.

Though they may appear outwardly strong and competent, agents are driven by an inner desperation to help others, often to the point of burnout. This is frequently the result of childhood patterns in which their needs were dismissed in favor of caring for a parent or another significant adult (Rosenberg and Kitaen-Morse, 2004b). In adult relationships, agents often gravitate toward people who need their support, forming imbalanced relationships that further drain their energy.

Over time, this constant caregiving without receiving emotional nourishment in return leads to physical and emotional distress. The more consistent the agency, the more somatic distress accumulates, eventually manifesting as physical illness (Levine, 2010).

Agency becomes the glue that holds old patterns and character styles firmly in place, making it difficult to break free. Agents often define themselves through their acts of service, feeling a void inside that they try to fill by caring for others. Yet, in doing so, they neglect their own needs, leaving them with a persistent sense of emptiness.

Quiz: What Is Your Attachment Style?

Understanding Your Relationship Patterns

Explore your personal inclinations and their impact on your relationships by assessing the following statements. Consider your behavior in romantic settings as you respond. Using the provided scale, when you are finished, add the numbers next to your response.

1. Becoming too emotionally close to my partner tends to make me uneasy.
   - Strongly agree (1)
   - Agree (2)
   - Neither agree nor disagree (3)
   - Disagree (4)
   - Strongly disagree (5)
2. Concerns about my partner's potential withdrawal of love are often on my mind.
   - Strongly agree (5)
   - Agree (4)
   - Neither agree nor disagree (3)

- Disagree (2)
- Strongly disagree (1)

3. Disagreements with my partner seldom prompt me to question the overall health of our relationship.
   - Strongly agree (1)
   - Agree (2)
   - Neither agree nor disagree (3)
   - Disagree (4)
   - Strongly disagree (5)

4. I hesitate to express my true feelings, fearing my partner might not reciprocate.
   - Strongly agree (5)
   - Agree (4)
   - Neither agree nor disagree (3)
   - Disagree (2)
   - Strongly disagree (1)

5. Offering emotional support during challenging times is something I find challenging.
   - Strongly agree (1)
   - Agree (2)
   - Neither agree nor disagree (3)
   - Disagree (4)
   - Strongly disagree (5)

6. I don't feel the need to introduce drama into my romantic relationships.
   - Strongly agree (1)
   - Agree (2)
   - Neither agree nor disagree (3)
   - Disagree (4)
   - Strongly disagree (5)

7. There's an underlying fear that others may not appreciate the real me once they get to know me.
   - Strongly agree (5)
   - Agree (4)
   - Neither agree nor disagree (3)
   - Disagree (2)

- Strongly disagree (1)

8. Independence holds greater significance for me than my relationships.
   - Strongly agree (1)
   - Agree (2)
   - Neither agree nor disagree (3)
   - Disagree (4)
   - Strongly disagree (5)

9. Providing natural comfort to my partner when upset is not one of my strengths.
   - Strongly agree (1)
   - Agree (2)
   - Neither agree nor disagree (3)
   - Disagree (4)
   - Strongly disagree (5)

10. In periods without a relationship, a sense of anxiety and incompleteness tends to set in.
    - Strongly agree (5)
    - Agree (4)
    - Neither agree nor disagree (3)
    - Disagree (2)
    - Strongly disagree (1)

11. Feeling that others depend on me is something I find distasteful.
    - Strongly agree (1)
    - Agree (2)
    - Neither agree nor disagree (3)
    - Disagree (4)
    - Strongly disagree (5)

12. Some might perceive me as predictable because I steer clear of unnecessary drama in relationships.
    - Strongly agree (1)
    - Agree (2)
    - Neither agree nor disagree (3)
    - Disagree (4)
    - Strongly disagree (5)

13. While I miss my partner during separations, a desire to escape arises when we reunite.
    - Strongly agree (1)
    - Agree (2)
    - Neither agree nor disagree (3)
    - Disagree (4)
    - Strongly disagree (5)

14. Expressing my needs and desires to my partner poses little difficulty for me.
    - Strongly agree (3)
    - Agree (2)
    - Neither agree nor disagree (1)
    - Disagree (4)
    - Strongly disagree (5)

15. If someone I'm dating becomes distant, concerns about potential wrongdoing on my part arise.
    - Strongly agree (5)
    - Agree (4)
    - Neither agree nor disagree (3)
    - Disagree (2)
    - Strongly disagree (1)

16. I tend to recover quickly after a breakup, effortlessly putting someone out of my mind.
    - Strongly agree (1)
    - Agree (2)
    - Neither agree nor disagree (3)
    - Disagree (4)
    - Strongly disagree (5)

17. There's a persistent worry that if my partner leaves, finding someone else might be challenging.
    - Strongly agree (5)
    - Agree (4)
    - Neither agree nor disagree (3)
    - Disagree (2)
    - Strongly disagree (1)

18. If someone I'm dating becomes distant, I may wonder about the cause but recognize it's likely not about me.
   - Strongly agree (1)
   - Agree (2)
   - Neither agree nor disagree (3)
   - Disagree (4)
   - Strongly disagree (5)

Scoring:

- Tally your points for each question.

Interpretation:

- **61–90 points:** Anxious Attachment Style
- **48–60 points:** Secure Attachment Style
- **18–47 points:** Avoidant Attachment Style

Art Directive: Mapping Past Relationships

Understanding and Navigating Patterns

This art directive invites you to reflect on past relationships, examining recurring patterns, how those relationships evolved or ended, the challenges that emerged, and the ways they provided support, stability, or feelings of rejection. While it's difficult to trace the exact origins of this directive or fully credit the Art Therapists who influenced its development, the work of **Monica Carpendale**, founder and former dean of the Kutenai Art Therapy Institute, and **Millie Cumming**, former dean of the Institute, have significantly shaped the approach I'm sharing here.

Materials Needed

- Large piece of white paper.
- Pencil crayons, markers, crayons, pencil(s) of your choosing.
- Any other artistic medium of your choosing including collage materials (optional).

Art Therapy Directive

- Allow yourself to take a few deep breaths to the ground, feeling your feet on the floor beneath you and feel yourself supported in a chair or sitting on the floor.
- Reflect on meaningful connections and relationships throughout your life who have had a significant impact, creating a mental inventory. These can include romantic, friendship, professional, or parental.
- Create a timeline on your page—this can be straight, curved, or any shape that feels right, guided by your own intuitive prompts felt in the body. Consider those you've connected with over the years, how these relationships have shaped you, and whether the experiences were positive, negative, or both. Use any imagery, symbols, or colors that come to mind to express these relationships and their influence on your personal journey.
- Map each relationship and connection (you could focus on just one type of relationship if you like, like romantic, friendship, etc.) on this timeline with a beginning, moving into the present. Notice any feelings that come up during this process as you continue adding relationships to your timeline and write these feelings down.
- Next to each relationship, include feelings, situations, or issues that you remember. You can write these out or express them with colors, collages, or any other means that feel appropriate.

If some relationships are too difficult to look at, note them on your timeline and move on. Take care of yourself in this moment, knowing that right now you are safe. Breathe into that space within you that holds the highest loving and supportive intention for your Soul's purpose. Feel this energy from within, filling you and surrounding you, helping you move through this process.

As you finish including all relationships that seem important, go back now, and reflect on what you may have learned from each relationship. Notice if you see any patterns in your relationship timeline. What would you like from future relationships that you may not have felt from the ones in your past? Include any new insights or feelings that have come up in your journal and be sure to date your page so you can look back at this exploration in the future.

Meditation to Heal Attachment Wounds

To Begin

Sit comfortably in an easy pose—either cross-legged on the floor or mat, or seated on a chair. Keep your eyes slightly open just a sliver, focusing gently on the **Third Eye Point**, located between your eyebrows. Rest your wrists on your knees with your hands in **Gyan Mudra**: touch the tips of your index fingers to your thumbs, while keeping the other fingers extended.

Mantra: SAA-TAA-NAA-MAA, RAA-MAA-DAA-SAA, SAA-SAY-SO-HUNG

Language: Sanskrit

Meaning:

- *Sa* (infinity)
- *Ta* (life)
- *Na* (death)
- *Ma* (rebirth)
- *Ra* (sun) – root chakra
- *Ma* (moon) – sacral chakra
- *Da* (earth) – navel chakra
- *Sa* (infinity) – heart and throat chakras
- *Sa, Say* (all that is infinity) – third eye chakra
- *So* (I am) – crown chakra
- *Hung* (the infinite) – sends energy from the crown back to the root chakra

Part I

- Chant the mantra on a single breath, as you press the fingertips sequentially with each syllable to the thumb starting with the pointer (Jupiter) finger, ending with the pinkie (mercury finger), and returning to the pointer finger as you continue. Use a mono-tone voice.

- Time: You may continue this meditation for 11 minutes or how-ever long you choose.

Part II

- Inhale deeply and suspend the breath. As you keep the breath held in, begin moving your body slowly as you twist and stretch. Move each muscle of the body; the head, torso, arms, back, belly, and hands. Then exhale powerfully through rounded lips.
- Repeat this 3–5 times.

Part III

- Immediately sit straight. Look at the tip of the nose and become totally calm and still.
- Meditate for 2–3 minutes.

To End

- Inhale and hold your breath for 30 seconds as you physically move and rotate your body as if it is going through spasms. Move and squeeze every muscle.
- Repeat this 3 more times.
- Then inhale, sit calmly, and concentrate on the tip of your nose for 20 seconds. Exhale and relax.

This meditation supports you in releasing and letting go of attachments that no longer serve you. It invites in a hopefulness for healthy new connections so you may live a fulfilled and joyful life.

As we let go of what no longer serves us, we create space energetically for what we want to come into our lives. Stay open to the possibilities as you release. Trust in your inner knowingness that healthy attachments are on their way.

Journaling and Reflections

In reading through the lessons for this module, you are invited to reflect in your journal on which attachment style you may relate to. Reflecting on your own childhood, take this moment of writing and reflection to notice how you were initially parented. How has this contributed to the way you are in relationships today? Allow any feelings to come up so they may be realized and moved if they cause discomfort. You are the adult now and have the power to love yourself in ways that will support your growth and journey.

In reading through the good parent messages, notice which ones feel true and which are more difficult to say to yourself or remember. Are there any that cause your attention to unconsciously wander off?

You are now an adult and have the power to become the parent you needed to feel secure in this world. It is not that our parents did a bad job necessarily, being a parent is a difficult and multilayered task. However, if you find that there were ways of being supported that were unavailable to you as a child, now is the time to fully embrace your inner child and offer that support that was not given.

Take this time to be quiet with yourself and listen to your body and any messages that may arise. Come back to your breathing and know that you are fully supported in this moment. You are caring for yourself in the ways you always needed.

Continuing Your 40-Day Practice

You have already moved into the sixth module of this program and had some time to begin your routine of a 40-day practice. Reflect on your own attachment style as you meditate. Has your awareness of where it originated given any deeper understanding?

If you've already reached 40 days, would you like to continue with this practice, or is there another you'd like to explore? Routine can give us a sense of control in our lives, and regular meditation supports the rerouting of neural pathways in the brain. Research highlights that mindfulness practices and consistent meditation help reshape the brain's patterns, improving emotional regulation and well-being (Davidson and McEwen, 2012). How have you noticed your life change since the beginning? Keep track of these changes in your journal as you move into the last modules of this program.

As described on page 136, ancient yogic teachings suggest that the number of days you commit to practice can significantly affect your habits and long-term well-being. Yogic tradition, similar to modern research on habit formation, suggests that consistent practice over specific time frames can break old habits and establish new patterns of behavior. In behavioral science, it is often highlighted that routine practices are critical in forming long-lasting habits (Clear, 2018). Here is a review of the yogic milestones you can aim for:

- **40 Days**: Practicing every day for 40 days straight will help break any negative habits that may block you from experiencing the full expansion that is possible through your meditation or mantra.
- **90 Days**: Practicing every day for 90 days straight will establish a new habit in your conscious and subconscious mind based on the effects of the meditation or mantra. You will notice significant changes during this time.
- **120 Days**: Practicing every day for 120 days straight will confirm the new habit of consciousness created by the meditation. The positive benefits of your practice will become integrated permanently into your psyche.
- **1000 Days**: Practicing every day for 1000 days straight will allow you to master your new habit of consciousness. No matter what challenges arise, you will be able to rely on this new habit to support you.

Reflect on where you are in your practice and consider continuing for a longer period if it feels aligned with your goals. Keep track of your progress in your journal, observing the subtle or significant changes over time. Consistent meditation has been shown to foster neuroplasticity, supporting the brain's ability to reorganize and form new neural connections, making lasting change possible (Davidson and McEwen, 2012).

Summary: Understanding Our Attachment Styles

Module Six focuses on the profound impact of early attachment patterns on emotional and psychological development, particularly in the context of psychedelic therapy. This module provides a framework for understanding and healing attachment related wounds, which is essential for achieving lasting inner awareness and emotional healing. Exploring attachment theory and inner child healing highlights how the bonds formed between children and their caregivers shape attachment styles—secure, anxious, avoidant, and disorganized—and how these patterns influence relationships and emotional resilience.

Key Support Elements for Your Journey:

1. **Integration in Psychedelic Therapy:**
   - **Exploration of Attachment Issues:** Psychedelic therapy provides profound emotional insights, bringing awareness to the roots of one's attachment style. Clients can confront and reprocess foundational experiences.
   - **Transformation of Attachment Patterns:** Insights from psychedelic experiences can be integrated into daily life, helping individuals develop more secure attachment behaviors, leading to healthier relationships and improved emotional regulation.

2. **Understanding Attachment Styles:**
   Anxious or Preoccupied Attachment Style:
   - Insecurity in relationships, constant worry about rejection, requiring constant reassurance, and high emotionality.
   - Fear, hurt, anger, and rejection from past issues intrude into present perceptions, leading to conflict and unpredictable moods.

   Avoidant, Dismissive, or Ambivalent Attachment Style:
   - Emotional distance, rejection of closeness, preference for autonomy, and non-emotional crisis handling.
   - Avoiding conflict and maintaining emotional independence, leading to disengaged and detached behavior.

   Secure Attachment Style:
   - Emotional closeness, safety, and comfort in relationships, easy communication, and emotional availability.
   - Trust, empathy, tolerance of differences, and balanced emotional state.

   Disorganized or Fearful-Avoidant Attachment Style:
   - Difficulty regulating emotions, quickness to anger, severe depression, PTSD symptoms, and dissociative habits.
   - Recreating past traumas in relationships, leading to abusive and dysfunctional patterns.

3. **What Creates Our Attachment Styles in Relationships:**
   Here we explore the reasons behind attachment patterns forming as they do. A look at the Primary Scenario of one's formative seven years is where much of our relationship styles are formed. This section highlights the need for living a fully embodied somatic life in order to become aware of feelings within relationships as we work towards a healthy attachment style.

4. **Good Parent Messages:**
   Early childhood messages are essential for developing a secure sense of self and attachment. These include affirmations of love, care, trust, and support.

5. **How Do Secure Attachment Patterns Develop:**
   Exploring ways one can move from anxious or avoidant attachment styles into secure and healthy patterns of connecting with others is addressed. Crucial for emotional stability are forming a bond with the primary caregiver, developing empathic attunement, and allowing sufficient space for a child to learn, experience, and express themselves.

6. **Quiz: What is Your Attachment Style:**
   A quiz to help individuals understand their attachment styles and how they impact relationships.

7. **Art Directive: Mapping Past Relationships:**
   An exercise to explore past relationships, identify patterns, and reflect on the support or rejection experienced.

8. **Meditation to Heal Attachment Wounds:**
   A meditation practice to release attachments that no longer serve and invite healthy new connections.

9. **Journaling and Reflections:**
   Reflect on personal attachment styles, childhood experiences, and the impact on current relationships. Embrace and support the inner child to foster growth and healing.

Understanding attachment styles is crucial for personal growth. The module invites you to explore your attachment patterns, recognize their impact on your relationships, and develop self-awareness to move beyond dysfunctional patterns. It provides tools and exercises, such as meditation and art directives, to support this process, fostering a more secure attachment style and enhancing emotional well-being. Through this exploration, you are encouraged to heal your own attachment wounds, embrace self-compassion, and cultivate healthier, more fulfilling relationships. This becomes pivotal as we move through the integration process and follow Judith Herman's (1992) stages of trauma therapy, although not concurrent, into the third stage and final stage.

Note

1. Good Parent Messages Retrieved from http://www.ibponline.org/resources/Couples_ Therapy.pdf, INTEGRATIVE BODY PSYCHOTHERAPY Sustaining Love and Sexuality in Long Term Intimate Relationships, Jack Lee Rosenberg, Ph.D., and Beverly Kitaen Morse, Ph.D.

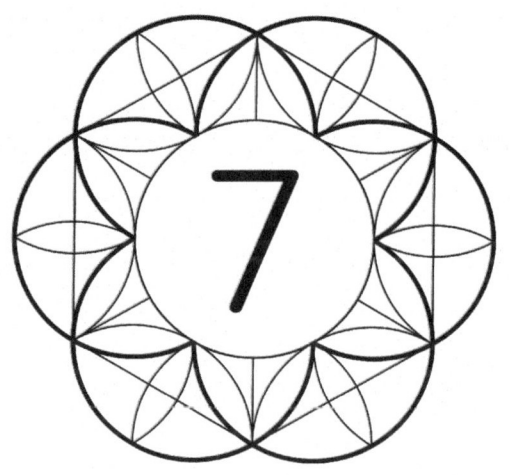

Module 7
Creating Healthy Connections

How We Can Connect in Healthy and Nourishing Ways

The final stage of trauma healing often centers on how we connect with others. This mirrors the three-stage model of trauma therapy, where after establishing safety and working through traumatic memories, the focus shifts to building relationships and fostering connections. This phase highlights that deep, lasting healing occurs when we can relate to others from a place of authenticity and self-acceptance (Herman, 1992).

Throughout the psychedelic integration process, you've been developing a relationship with your experience and the transformation it has sparked within you. Now, it's time to look outward—to examine the ways you connect with others and strengthen your social bonds. Building healthy connections is a critical aspect of growth and self-acceptance. The ability to engage with others from a place of openness, without over-relying on others or shutting yourself off, is a significant marker of emotional healing (Harris, 2015).

A measurement of true healing can be seen in how we reach out for support. This module invites you to reflect on your patterns. Do you reach out for help when needed? Do you shut people out and over-rely on yourself? Or do you merge with others to the point that you struggle to distinguish your emotions from theirs (Johnson, 2008)? Balancing these

　　　　DOI: 10.4324/9781003595762-26

dynamics is key, and building strong, flexible boundaries is essential to nurturing healthy, interdependent relationships (Brown, 2017).

Just as we need a balanced diet for physical health, our relationships also require balance. You wouldn't seek a dentist for a broken leg, and in the same way, we must recognize the unique roles that different relationships play in our lives. Consider how you can meet different emotional needs through different relationships and maintain boundaries that ensure healthy dynamics with the people around you (Neff, 2011). Identifying where different people can support you—and where they cannot— creates more realistic expectations and fosters growth in all connections.

There is wisdom in the saying, "The other person is you." People often act as mirrors, reflecting parts of ourselves that we may love or, in some cases, wish to change. Relationships offer the opportunity to work through these reflections, making them a key part of the integration process. By connecting with others, we gain deeper awareness and compassion, both for ourselves and those around us (Siegel, 2012).

In the final stages of integration, connecting with others who have shared similar experiences can provide invaluable support. Whether it's through online groups, local communities, or shared spaces dedicated to psychedelic experiences, reaching out to others can help cement the transformation you've experienced. Consider making a list of places or people you feel drawn to, even if you don't act on it right away. You can brainstorm ways to foster these connections when the time feels right.

By allowing yourself to be seen by others—within healthy, supportive boundaries—you continue moving toward a life filled with joy, connection, and self-acceptance. This is the culmination of the integration process, where you can live in the fullness of your being, free from the constraints of fear, shame, or isolation.

Boundaries and How They Are Created

What are boundaries, and how does having—or not having—them affect our lives? Where are these "boundaries" formed, and why do we need them? Boundaries are crucial in understanding how we connect with others, whether they serve as protective mechanisms or create obstacles. The type of boundaries we hold often connects directly to our attachment style. For instance, those with avoidant attachment styles may have more rigid boundaries, while those with anxious attachment styles tend to have softer, more diffuse boundaries (Levine and Heller, 2010).

Boundaries are developed as coping mechanisms in response to our early life experiences. When we enter the world, we are open, with a clear sense of Self. However, over time, through experiences and life events, we learn to protect ourselves. This protection may manifest as personality traits, ways of reacting, or methods of interaction, such as keeping people at a distance or, conversely, enmeshing ourselves with others and losing our sense of individuality (Siegel, 2012). The work we are doing here is to open up, allowing our true Self to shine through, all while maintaining an understanding of the importance of healthy boundaries.

Within a human connection, there is always an energetic exchange. Have you ever been in the presence of someone who talks endlessly about their life, leaving you drained afterward? Or have you ever noticed someone enter a room, and the energy of the space shifts, for better or worse? Energy plays a crucial role in how we connect and affect one another (Rosenberg and Kitaen-Morse, 2004a). Recognizing this dynamic and learning how to manage our energy—whether it's sharing it or protecting it—is at the heart of this module.

By developing the skills to recognize and modify your boundaries, you enhance your ability to connect with others authentically and intimately. This process can be thought of as "energetic hygiene"—just as we need to care for our physical bodies, we must also care for the energy we bring into and take from relationships (Goleman, 2006). Learning to say no when necessary or yes when we genuinely feel ready becomes part of this important work.

One method for strengthening and becoming more aware of your boundaries is through meditation. Envision yourself surrounded by a light that gives you the space to be yourself while protecting you from energies that don't serve you. Begin consciously choosing whom you let into this energetic space. This practice connects back to earlier discussions on aura-strengthening techniques, which are essential for maintaining energetic boundaries (Judith, 2001).

The way we form boundaries is heavily influenced by our attachment patterns. As we discussed earlier, the manner in which we connect or avoid connection can greatly affect our relationships. One key to understanding ourselves through the lens of attachment is examining how our boundaries have been formed and recognizing the reasons behind their creation (Bowlby, 1988).

As we explore these areas, it's essential to suspend judgment. Nothing is inherently right or wrong. Our boundaries, and the way we interact with the world, have been developed to maximize safety. The human psyche is remarkably adept at creating strategies for survival (Schore, 2003). While these strategies may have been necessary in childhood, they often continue into adulthood when they're no longer useful. By moving toward a more secure attachment style, we can break free from these old patterns and develop relationships that are safe, fulfilling, and nourishing (Siegel, 2012).

Boundaries are not barriers. They aren't meant to keep others out or to keep us locked in. Instead, they allow us to feel safe in relationships and to navigate the world meaningfully, connecting with others without fear of rejection or judgment. This process doesn't happen overnight. But by reflecting on the way we connect with others and adjusting our boundaries, we open ourselves to more love and connection.

So, how do we get there? How do we find the perfect balance between being too open or too closed off? It starts by recognizing what was missing during our upbringing and working to repair that through self-parenting (Schwartz, 2020b). Healing the inner child is often a deep and difficult process, but connecting to the strengths and resources you've cultivated throughout this program is key. Create a space—both physically and emotionally—where you can express those unmet childhood needs. This space represents a boundary in itself, reminding you that you deserve time and care.

Inner Child Healing

The work of acknowledging and reparenting your inner child is a crucial step toward creating the ability to safely reach out to others. This process involves reconnecting with and healing the child-like aspects of the psyche that may have been neglected or wounded during childhood. Reparenting oneself fosters a secure attachment style, which enables healthier, more fulfilling relationships with others.

At its core, inner child work addresses unresolved emotions and traumas from one's formative years. These early experiences can still influence adult behaviors, emotional responses, and even relationship patterns (Siegel, 2012). By developing a relationship with your inner child, you can address the ways it continues to act out the "old story"—whether that involves feeling unsupported, abandoned, or controlled in childhood. As your inner child begins to feel safer in the world and trusts that the adult part of you will provide care, a more integrated and balanced sense of self can emerge (Schwartz, 2020b).

One of the most essential parts of reparenting is learning to cultivate self-compassion. Often, this is easier said than done, especially for those who may not have experienced unconditional love in childhood. However, if you imagine yourself as a young child—an innocent, curious, and vulnerable being—it may be easier to tap into that sense of compassion. What did this young version of you need most? Imagining yourself with the same love you would offer a small child can be transformative (Brown, 2020). This perspective shift helps in nurturing the self-compassion required to heal emotional wounds.

Psychedelic experiences often facilitate powerful emotional engagement with the inner child. Psychedelics can bring symbolic representations of one's childhood to the forefront, providing an opportunity to re-experience early life events or relational wounds with a fresh perspective (Carhart-Harris and Friston, 2019). Such encounters may allow for profound emotional release, personal growth, and an improved sense of connection with oneself and others. These experiences, when properly integrated, can lead to a more profound sense of emotional security and self-acceptance.

Throughout this module, we will explore ways to reconnect with your inner child and recognize when it needs support. By doing this, you will build the necessary foundation for greater emotional resilience and healthier relationships moving forward.

Experiential: Supporting Your Inner Child

An Exercise to Create Self-Love, Support and Healing

Recommendations: If at any point during this directive, you begin to feel unsafe, notice your feet on the ground. Press into them and bring yourself back into the present moment with full belly breaths. Look around the room and name ten items around you and their color.

Supporting Your Inner Child

If it feels safe, imagine yourself now as a child. What age comes up first for you? Notice how you feel at this age. Is there anything you need? Is there anything you remember not having or maybe having too much of?

It can be a bit overwhelming to revisit the past but take comfort in knowing that right now, your inner child is safe. In this moment, you're fully immersed in something that brings you joy and fills you with fun. As you take in your surroundings, you realize you're in a place that feels both safe and comforting. Then, you spot your adult self approaching. Curiosity stirs inside you, and with growing excitement, you feel a wave of happiness. This moment fills you with warmth and security. While there might have been times when things felt uncertain or frightening, right now, you're a child, experiencing pure joy in a safe, warm, and welcoming space. Let yourself fully embrace that feeling. Breathe into this sense of safety and comfort, and notice how it feels in your body.

Now, imagine yourself as the adult you are in this present moment, watching this child and witnessing those earlier versions of yourself with complete happiness. You feel such tremendous warmth towards the child and feel such warm love *from* this child. You reach out to the child and ask if they would like a hug. If they agree, bring them in close and feel their love as you merge the love you have for this innocent child. If coming close doesn't feel comfortable for your inner child, let them know that that is okay too. Let them know that everything is good and that they are loved and cared for.

As you wrap your arms around this young version of you or sit with them holding space, allow whatever feelings that may arise to come to the surface for both of you. Allow any pain to surface, knowing that at this moment you are the adult and helping to heal a side of yourself that was unable to access this comfort in this particular way. You are the parent now. Porges' (2011) polyvagal theory underscores the importance of creating safety and connection to facilitate emotional regulation and healing, which is especially relevant to this exercise of inner child work. Breathe with a full cleansing breath, imagining any stress leaving your body with the exhale, moving it into the earth where it will be cleansed.

Ask your inner child if they would like to come with you now, imagining a place that brings you comfort and safety in the present. Bring your inner child with you to this place if they are open to coming. If not, they can choose to stay where they are, and you can remind them that you will continue to look out for them and protect them. If your child decides to come with you, place them in this safe place, and let them know that you will continue to care for them and watch over them. Whatever they may have felt scared of is now gone, and they are protected and loved completely, unconditionally.

Let them know that they can call on you whenever needed, asking them in this moment how they would like to connect. Maybe it is a feeling you will receive within your body? Maybe a thought will come to mind, and you will know this is them needing your support and comfort. Just stay open to whatever message they would like you to receive, for you to know they need you. Siegel (2012) speaks to the profound impact of mindfulness and attachment-focused work on neuroplasticity, suggesting that healing occurs when we stay open to these inner communications. Assure them that you are an adult now and can support them in ways they may not have felt in the past.

Now may be a good time to tap into the healing you felt during your non-ordinary state experience. Was there a presence you remember that was guiding you and supporting you? You may understand this energetic force to have come from within you, from outside of you as a separate being or spirit, or the spirit of the medicine. Breathe into this energy and ask it in this moment to return and hold you as you hold the younger version of you from the past. Stay open to any messages that may come forward from the energy or spirit/being of your mystical experience and from your inner child. Ask your inner child what it needs in this moment and imagine yourself giving that to them now. Feel the adult version of you holding, loving, and healing the inner child in you who has needed this support for so long.

Staying with your breath and the experience, when you are ready to come back into the room, grab your journal and begin writing any feelings out and draw or color any images that come to you. You may even invite the child within you to color and create what they would like to show you.

Finally, continue moving this healing energy through your body. Recognize the capacity for growth that you hold. This is deep work, and you are making tremendous progress. Remember, you can return to this exercise whenever you feel the need for extra support or when you recognize old coping patterns that no longer serve you. Schwartz (2020a) highlights that Inner Child work, when aligned with self-energy, leads to profound shifts in healing and self-compassion.

Reparenting Ourselves

Moving Into Secure Attachment

Feeling secure in the way we connect with others helps create harmonious and balanced relationships and friendships. In this section, we will explore what is needed to shift towards a more secure attachment style. As mentioned earlier, attachment styles are developed largely in the first seven years of life and are shaped by our relationships with caregivers or parents (Bowlby, 1988; Schore, 2003). When disruptions occur during this period, we, as adults, are often left to re-parent our inner child and find healthier ways to nurture ourselves—especially when old wounds are triggered in relationships. It is in the context of relationships that we can best identify what triggers us into old patterns. Recognizing these attachment patterns brings us into the present moment and helps us learn how to halt behaviors that have become so familiar.

What Is a Secure Attachment Pattern?

- **Comfortable being close and affectionate with others but also okay with being alone**: People with secure attachment feel balanced in their ability to connect and detach healthily (Siegel, 2012). They are not overly dependent on others for validation and enjoy time alone without feeling abandoned.
- **Able to openly communicate your needs and also cater to the needs of your partner**: Secure attachment allows individuals to express their needs openly while also being sensitive to the needs of others. They avoid manipulation or game-playing in relationships (Johnson, 2008).
- **Positive beliefs about others' intentions**: Securely attached people tend to have more positive views of others and expect their

relationships to be mutually supportive, rather than suspicious or distrustful (Shaver and Mikulincer, 2012).

- **Able to handle rejection well and not play games**: Rejection or conflict does not significantly shake the sense of self in securely attached individuals. They are more resilient, can tolerate disappointment, and do not retaliate by playing emotional games (Hazan and Shaver, 1987).
- **Can engage in healthy conflict, without causing insult or injury**: Conflict is seen as a normal part of relationships for those with secure attachment, and they are capable of navigating it in a way that preserves respect for both themselves and their partners (Siegel, 2012).
- **Expect good things to happen to you and believe that you are worthy of this**: Secure attachment fosters self-worth and an expectation that positive experiences are deserved, reinforcing an overall optimistic view of relationships (Schore, 2003).
- **Well-developed instincts around relationships—you know when a relationship is no longer healthy and will act on this**: Secure attachment enables individuals to trust their instincts about when a relationship is becoming harmful or unhealthy and to take action to protect themselves (Johnson, 2008).

Rewiring Your Attachment Style

Effective Ways to Support Growth and Change

Reparenting ourselves to achieve a Secure Attachment style requires acknowledging our triggers and having compassion for where these reactions originated. This self-awareness helps us navigate relationships with greater ease and emotional balance. Moving towards secure attachment is a journey, and it's essential to treat yourself with the same kindness and patience you would show a small child learning something new. Below are some key steps to rewiring your attachment style and supporting personal growth:

1. **What Do You Love Doing? Do it More!** Living passionately involves cultivating activities that bring you joy and fulfillment.

These are the things you're naturally good at, that bring a sense of accomplishment, and that allow you to enter a state of flow. Make time each week to deepen your connection to these activities. Passionate living is a key step toward feeling confident and secure in yourself (Brown, 2010).

If you're unsure what your passions are, write a list of activities that spark joy, and dedicate time each day or week to explore them. Often, we discover what we're passionate about by stumbling upon it, realizing we're fully absorbed and in our element. It's a gift to take time for yourself to explore these moments (Csikszentmihalyi, 1990).

2. **Push Yourself Out of Your Comfort Zone:** Building self-esteem involves facing fears and stepping into uncomfortable situations. Write down areas of your life that make you feel uneasy—nothing dangerous, just things that challenge your routine. Choose one or two to focus on and consciously push yourself in a safe, manageable way. Personal growth requires courage, and with each challenge, you'll discover strengths you didn't know you had (Bowlby, 1988; Siegel, 2012).

3. **Strengthen Your Body Physically:** Physical well-being supports emotional and mental resilience. Start small but make an effort to engage in some form of physical activity daily. Whether it's a short walk, yoga, or weight training, nurturing your physical body helps develop a sense of emotional stability and strength (Levine, 2010).

4. **Create a Deeper Sense of Self-Compassion:** Often, we're our own worst critics. Start by becoming aware of how you speak to yourself. If your inner voice is harsh, critical, or unkind, ask yourself if you would speak to a child that way. Self-compassion involves treating yourself with the same kindness you would extend to others. This mindset shift can transform how you relate to yourself and others (Neff, 2011).

5. **Insight, Understanding, and Awareness Generate Emotional Freedom:** Insight helps you understand why certain patterns repeat in your life and relationships. It's not about making excuses,

but about understanding the roots of your behaviors and reactions so you can stop them from controlling your future. When you feel a reaction brewing—whether it's pushing someone away or clinging to them—pause and ask yourself, *Why?* Cultivating self-awareness creates space for healthier responses (Schore, 2003).

6. **Focus on Healing:** Childhood traumas often lead to shame, low self-esteem, and insecure attachment styles. Healing these wounds allows you to build the foundation for secure attachments. Begin by addressing feelings of shame, self-neglect, and self-sabotage, and work towards letting go of self-doubt (Brown, 2010).

7. **Build Self-Esteem:** Once you've started healing, it's time to build your sense of self-worth. Forgive yourself for past mistakes, let go of shame, and begin the process of positive self-talk and self-acceptance. Building self-esteem takes time, but it's essential for creating secure, loving relationships (Neff, 2011).

8. **Communicate Your Needs:** In healthy relationships, clear communication is key. Don't be afraid to express what you need. Instead of focusing on what your partner isn't doing, articulate how you would like things to change to feel more supported, loved, and connected. Open dialogue helps deepen emotional intimacy (Siegel, 2012).

9. **Learn How to Handle Conflict Effectively:** Conflict isn't the end of a relationship—it's an opportunity to grow closer. Be open about your fears and concerns, and don't avoid difficult conversations. Avoidant individuals often fear conflict, but facing it head-on allows for greater intimacy and trust. Avoid assumptions; always ask for clarification to strengthen your relationship (Johnson, 2008).

10. **Shift from Self-Reliance to Mutual Support:** In secure relationships, both partners should feel supported and able to depend on each other. Letting go of self-reliance can be difficult, especially if past experiences have led you to believe you can't trust others. However, relying on each other fosters mutual respect, intimacy, and trust (Bowlby, 1988).

Art Directive: Inside Outside Box
What We Share and What We Do Not

In this module, we will delve deeper into the ways we connect with others and how we present ourselves to the world. By exploring the contrast between how we feel inside and how we believe others perceive us, or how we want to be seen, we can bring greater awareness to our own authenticity. Often, we adapt ourselves to fit into our environment, but this exercise helps us become more aware of when and how this happens. Through this practice, we will aim to align our inner self with how we present externally, creating a more congruent and self-accepting existence—recognizing the divine perfection within us.

In this art directive, found in *Essence and Praxis in the Art Therapy Studio* (Carpendale, 2009, pp. 92–95), you will use a box and collage materials to visually represent this interplay. The inside of the box will reflect how you personally see yourself or feel within, while the outside will show how you think others perceive you or how you would like to be perceived. This directive offers a meaningful opportunity to reflect on how we show up in the world, what we may choose to keep hidden, and how we can integrate these two facets to embrace our authentic selves.

Research shows that externalizing internal feelings, such as through art-making, can support emotional processing and self-reflection (Malchiodi, 2015). Art Therapy, particularly in expressive modalities like collage, has been widely recognized for its ability to provide insight into inner emotional states and to foster greater self-awareness (Moon, 2002a). These artistic processes can help facilitate a clearer understanding of the self, both as seen internally and projected externally, contributing to deeper personal integration (Schore, 2003).

Materials Needed:

- Glue stick or glue bottle (a glue stick works well for collage images).
- Scissors.
- Miscellaneous materials such as yarn, buttons, shells, if desired.
- A box of your choice, with or without a lid (preferably large enough to display multiple images).

- Collage images from magazines, ads, or printed from online sources. Begin cutting out images intuitively; don't overthink which images to collect—trust that the ones you are drawn to have meaning.

Steps to Begin:

1. **Create Your Space**

   Find a comfortable art space where you feel safe and can work uninterrupted. If you've already started gathering collage materials, you can bring them to your workspace, or begin collecting new images.

2. **Grounding in Breath**

   Begin by noticing your breath. If you feel comfortable, close your eyes. Expand your breath slowly, filling your belly, lungs, side ribs, and up to your clavicle before gently releasing it. Notice any sensations in your body as you exhale, releasing all air before the next inhale.

   If any discomfort arises in your body, breathe into that space, allowing the exhale to release tension. Continue to ground yourself, feeling the support beneath you as your breath expands and your body settles.

3. **Tuning into Your Inner Knowing**

   As you deepen your breath, focus your awareness on the part of you that holds your inner wisdom—your essence, spirit, or Soul. Breathe into this space and feel it expand through your body. Stay present with your breath and your inner knowing.

4. **Selecting Collage Images**

   When you feel ready, open your eyes and begin selecting images for your collage. These images should represent how you feel inside and how you believe others see you, or how you wish to be seen. Trust your intuition. Even if an image doesn't immediately make sense, choose it—your inner knowing is guiding you, and the meaning will reveal itself as you work.

   According to Siegel (2012), using creative expression allows for accessing parts of the unconscious, which helps individuals articulate feelings and perceptions that might otherwise remain hidden. This process encourages a reflective practice, linking emotional experiences with conscious awareness.

5. **Assembling the Inside of the Box**

Begin by gluing the images that represent how you see yourself inside the box. This may evoke emotions, especially if there is a disconnect between what you hide and what you show. Allow any feelings to surface and know that you are held in a safe space as this shift takes place.

6. **Decorating the Outside of the Box**

Now, move to the outside of your box. Place images that represent how you think others perceive you or how you choose to present yourself to the world. Feel free to use other materials such as yarn, buttons, or shells to embellish the outside of your box, using a hot glue gun for heavier objects if necessary.

7. **Reflection**

As you finish, take time to sit with the emotions and thoughts that have surfaced during the process. Reflect on any disconnects between your inner self and outer presentation, and explore how you might bring these aspects into greater alignment. Journaling or drawing about the insights gained during this activity can also enhance self-awareness and emotional growth (Cameron, 1992). Move onto the next section now to read more on journaling, where you will be invited to write about or discuss the new understandings that have emerged, noting how this greater understanding of self-expression might influence your interactions moving forward.

Journaling

Once you have completed your Inside/Outside Box, take a pause, breathe deeply, and reflect using your journal. Journaling provides the space to process the feelings and insights that arise from this exercise, helping to deepen self-awareness and integrate the emotional experience into your conscious mind (Adams, 2016). Sit with your creation, stay connected to your breath, and notice how you feel as you contemplate what the box represents. Are there any shifts or insights that surface?

Begin by writing about the emotions or sensations that arose during the creation of your box:

- How do you see yourself on the inside compared to how others see you or how you present yourself to the world?
- Is there a disconnect between your inner self and outer expression? If so, why do you think this exists?
- Are there parts of you that feel safer being kept private? Reflect on what parts of your inner self you feel hesitant or unable to reveal.
- Are there parts of your external self that don't feel in alignment with your true nature or authentic self?
- What keeps you from showing more of your authentic self to others?

As you answer these questions, try to identify if there's a desire or need for greater alignment between your inner and outer worlds. According to Siegel (2012), integrating one's inner experiences with outer expressions is a core aspect of emotional regulation and authenticity, promoting a more balanced and harmonious life.

There might be very legitimate reasons to keep certain aspects of yourself private, but sometimes the act of naming these reasons can bring about shifts in how you show up in the world. At times, simply acknowledging why you hold back can create an opportunity for change or a deeper validation of your need for protection (Neff, 2011). Whatever the case may be, write these insights down and allow yourself the freedom to explore them in your journal.

When you finish journaling, you might want to name your box. Titles can help solidify the meaning of your artwork and give it a sense of completion. Place your box in a safe and visible place where it can serve as a reminder of the work you are doing.

With a final deep breath, acknowledge the journey you've undertaken with this exercise. Allow yourself to notice if there has been a shift—has this process led to a new or deeper awareness of yourself? Journaling, combined with creative expression, offers a powerful way to process and transform internal conflicts into conscious awareness (Carpendale, 2009).

Meditation: Sensing and Strengthening Your Boundaries

In this exercise, we'll explore the concept of boundaries, both physically and emotionally, through a meditative practice designed for two people. This practice allows for a deeper exploration of personal space and boundaries as a felt experience in the body. By engaging in this activity, you will gain insight into how boundaries affect interpersonal relationships, fostering self-awareness and comfort in maintaining them.

Instructions:

1. **Sit with your partner:** Begin by sitting across from another person on the floor. Take a moment to notice how the physical presence of the other person affects your body. What sensations do you feel? This could be subtle tension, ease, or perhaps neutrality.

2. **Create a boundary:** Using chalk, yarn, string, or another marker, draw a circle around yourself. This represents your personal boundary. As you do this, notice the size of the circle you're creating. Does it feel like the right size for you? Do you need more or less space? Adjust the boundary until it feels "just right."

3. **Make a boundary statement:** Communicate to the other person, saying something like, "This is my space. Please respect it unless I invite you in." Pay attention to how this makes you feel. Does asserting your boundary brings up feelings of discomfort or empowerment?

4. **Observe your partner's boundary:** Now, have the other person create their own boundary. As they do this, notice any changes in your body or feelings that arise. How do you perceive the contact between you? Are your boundaries touching, distant, or overlapping? Have them recite a boundary statement and notice how this feels for you to hear.

5. **Experiment with the boundary:** Play with the idea of proximity. Move closer to each other and allow your boundaries to overlap. How does this feel? Are you comfortable or uncomfortable with the overlap? Notice what happens emotionally and physically.

6. **Remove the boundary:** Once you've completed the exercise, slowly remove your boundary. Take time to observe how this

affects your internal experience. How does it feel to be without a boundary while sitting across from someone who still has one? Does this experience remind you of any past interactions with people in your life?

This exercise is designed to help participants become aware of their boundaries in interpersonal relationships. Many people find that creating boundaries enhances the sense of security and fosters healthier connections. The other person is no longer experienced as an extension of oneself, but as a separate individual with whom one can connect without losing one's sense of self.

For some individuals, particularly those with a fear of abandonment, creating a boundary may bring up fears of isolation or loneliness (Holmes, 2014). On the other hand, individuals with a fear of being engulfed by others may prefer to create multiple layers of boundaries as a form of protection (Schore, 2003). This variation in boundary-setting is often closely tied to one's attachment style, influencing how one perceives closeness and space in relationships (Bowlby, 1988).

This practice not only fosters self-awareness but also encourages a deeper understanding of the balance between maintaining personal space and fostering meaningful connections with others (Siegel, 2012).

Journaling and Reflections

Expanding Your Meditation and Art Making to Dive Deeper

After completing this module, take a moment to observe how you feel. Working on deep emotional topics such as reparenting the inner child, establishing healthy boundaries, and reflecting on how we connect with others can stir up emotions from the past. These emotions might bring up a range of feelings that require your attention and self-care.

Self-Care Reflection

In times of emotional vulnerability, it is crucial to prioritize self-care. I encourage you to take out your journal and list regular self-care practices that support you. Whether it is meditation, physical activity, time spent in nature, or connecting with loved ones, writing these practices down serves as a reminder of how to replenish your internal reserves when necessary. Research supports the importance of self-care in maintaining emotional resilience, particularly when engaging with therapeutic or personal development work (Neff, 2011; Siegel, 2010).

Journal Prompts for Reflection

If you have not been journaling consistently throughout this module, now is a great time to look back on the content you have covered. Review the module titles or key themes to identify any lingering questions or emotions that need to be addressed. Journaling can help you process these insights and consolidate any growth or healing you've experienced (Pennebaker, 1997). Here are a few prompts to help you get started:

- What emotions came up for me during this module? How did I handle them?
- Are there any parts of my inner child that still need nurturing?
- What boundaries do I feel more comfortable with now? Are there any boundaries I need to reassess?
- How has my understanding of my attachment style evolved throughout this module?
- What self-care practices have been most supportive to me during this process?

Journaling provides a space to expand upon the insights gained through meditation and creative exercises. This reflective process can help integrate your emotional experiences, deepening your understanding of yourself and your relationships (Schore, 2003).

Continuing Your 40-Day Practice

Here we are in the seventh module of this program. If you have been engaging in a 40-day practice, reflect back to when you first began and acknowledge the accomplishment of where you are now. Reflect on any transformations or ways you feel life has been shifting. The practice of regular meditation is a large part of truly integrating the effects of a psychedelic experience, as you develop healthy and sustained ways of fully being in the world.

Have you been able to share your experience of meditation with another? Maybe encourage someone you care about to join you in your commitment. Looking for other meditations to explore may be supportive as well. As you continue to safely connect to the community, maybe there is a regular meditation group that meets? Notice what feels right for you as you continue your journey by making meditation a regular part of your world.

Summary: Creating Healthy Connections

In Module Seven, we explore the final stage of trauma therapy, which emphasizes connecting to others as a path to lasting healing. Having established safety through the process of integrating the psychedelic experience, this module focuses on developing tools and strengths to form meaningful and nourishing relationships. The journey centers on sharing our lives with the world in ways that embody meaning, purpose, and self-acceptance.

Key Support Elements for Your Journey:

1. **How We Can Connect in Healthy and Nourishing Ways:**
   This section discusses the importance of forming healthy connections as the final stage of trauma therapy. It emphasizes self-acceptance as the foundation for these connections and encourages individuals to reflect on how they reach out to others and the quality of their relationships.

2. **Boundaries and How They are Created:**
   This part explores the significance of boundaries in relationships. It looks at how boundaries are formed, their role in maintaining healthy connections, and how they relate to different attachment styles. The section also discusses the balance between having too rigid or too diffuse boundaries and how they form.

3. **Inner Child Healing:**
   Inner child healing is highlighted as a crucial component of developing secure attachments. This section discusses reconnecting with and healing the wounded aspects of the psyche from childhood. It emphasizes the importance of reparenting oneself to create safety and security in adult relationships.

4. **Reparenting Ourselves:**

   Building on inner child work, this section delves into the process of reparenting. It focuses on developing a secure attachment style by addressing unresolved childhood traumas and fostering self-compassion, self-esteem, and emotional security.

5. **Rewiring Your Attachment Style:**

   Practical steps are offered here to help you move towards a secure attachment style. This includes strategies for building self-esteem, handling conflict, and improving communication in relationships. The section also stresses the importance of balancing self-reliance with mutual support in relationships.

6. **Art Directive: Inside Outside Box:**

   This creative exercise invites individuals to explore the disparity between their internal self-perception and how they are perceived by others. It also speaks to boundaries around what we share with the world, and what we keep close. Through art, one can reflect on inner feelings and how they choose to present themselves to the world, aiming to achieve greater congruence between the two.

7. **Meditation: Sensing and Strengthening Your Boundaries:**

   A mindfulness practice using string to somatically experience, and become more aware of your boundaries. This exercise is designed to enhance the felt sense of personal boundaries and experiment with how these boundaries affect interactions with others.

8. **Journaling and Reflections:**

   The final section encourages participants to reflect on their experiences throughout the module. Journaling is suggested as a tool for deepening self-awareness and processing emotions that arise from working on boundaries, inner child healing, and attachment styles. It also supports the ongoing integration of insights gained from the module.

9. **Continuing Your 40-day Practice:**

   As we move into this seventh chapter, you are invited to share your experience of regular meditation with others. With the theme of this chapter being connecting to others, working towards creating a community with meditation routines is encouraged.

The module offers practical exercises, including meditation and art directives, to help you explore your inner and outer self, recognize boundaries, and develop authentic connections. Through these practices, you are encouraged to integrate your mystical experience into your daily life and strengthen your ability to form healthy, supportive relationships. The ultimate goal is to create connections that are grounded in self-awareness, acceptance, and mutual respect, leading to a more fulfilling and harmonious life.

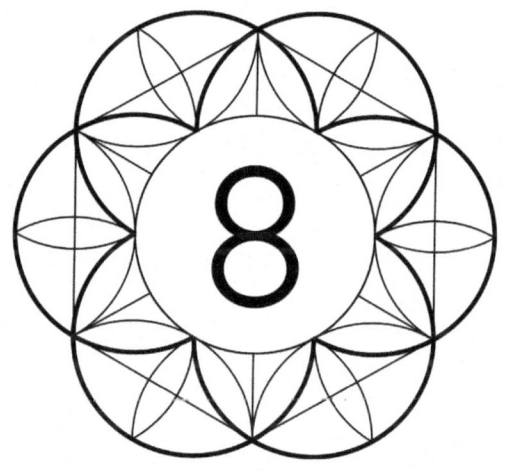

MODULE 8
INTEGRATING OUR SHADOW SIDE

Getting to Know and Love Your Shadow

From movements working to close the gap between rich and poor, to ending systemic racism, and supporting gender equality, we are learning every day about the lives of others with whom we share this planet. There is an unveiling happening in our world, and it feels more intense than ever. Some call this the Aquarian Age, while others reference prophecies that speak of Maya (the material world) dissolving to reveal only what is true (Bradford, 2020; Campbell, 2016). Globally, the unconscious is being made conscious, which can be an uncomfortable transition. How has this been for you?

It is within the unconscious that shadows live, and Psychedelics can serve as potent catalysts for bringing these shadow parts to the surface. Although it may feel uncomfortable, when shadow aspects are ready to emerge, they offer an opportunity for release and integration (Jung, 1969c; Grof, 1985). When these shadows can be seen, acknowledged, and given a voice, their hold on us begins to diminish. This is the core of Shadow Work.

However, our personal veils keep us feeling protected, and lifting them is no light and airy task. When parts of ourselves are hidden, filled with shame, judgment, and suppressed for too long, they begin to leak out in

 DOI: 10.4324/9781003595762-27

ways that do not serve our highest expression of Self. They morph into what we may describe as traits or parts of our personality, like shame, insecurities, judgments of others and ourselves, self-loathing, indecisiveness, and even depression and anxiety (Ford, 2017). The list can go on and on.

It's essential that we learn to accept our imperfections, acknowledging them as integral to who we are. Being perfect at everything would make us less human. Yet, society imposes standards, and we make judgments about what we should be, leading us to hide parts of ourselves (Bradford, 2020).

In this module, we focus on bringing these aspects into conscious awareness, integrating them in a way that diminishes their intensity, so they no longer control us. Often, we are unaware of these shadows, but working with them after a Non-Ordinary State of Consciousness (NOSC) experience can be one of the most transformative parts of the integration process (Grof, 1985).

You are invited to release what no longer serves you. Reflect on where these parts may have originated, and ask yourself what they need to express. If it feels safe, imagine them moving visibly into the light. If this feels too risky, express them through art or meditation. Remember, your psyche will only bring up what you are capable of handling in this moment. Trust that your Soul has guided you here and you possess the strength to move beyond what no longer serves you (Jung, 1969; Ford, 2017).

Jungian Psychology

Let's explore what the shadow is according to Carl Jung. In Jungian psychology, the shadow refers to the unconscious aspects of the personality that the conscious ego rejects. These are often the least desirable parts of ourselves, and so our conscious mind pushes them into the subconscious (Jung, 1938).

The more we push away these "negative" parts without giving them healthy outlets, the more destructive they become (Jung, 1953). These undesirable parts of the self can create chronic depression, addiction, or deep internalized resentment. Art, as a form of expression, can be an evocative and effective way to explore shadow aspects of ourselves (Moon, 2002a). Ground yourself during this process and know that you are safe as you engage in this work.

Practical Skills to Develop:

1. Stop labeling your weaknesses as problems.
2. Kindly accept them as parts of you, much like accepting a scar.
3. Say to yourself, "I accept all parts of me. Nothing is inherently good or bad; only thinking makes it so."
4. Stop striving for perfection. Ask yourself why you feel the need to be perfect.
5. Reflect on when you first learned this pattern.

Jungian Definitions that May Resonate with Your Experiences:

- **Authentic Self:** The true projection of your Soul. It is when we are intuitive and live in the experience of each moment.
- **Persona:** A projection from the authentic Self, but only the side we wish to show others.
- **Shadow Self:** The opposite of the Persona, the weaknesses we do not want to show. Accepting the Shadow makes us whole (Jung, 1953).
- **Hidden Self:** A false self-based on unresolved traumas from childhood. It blocks the natural radiance of the authentic Self.
- **Mask:** A projection of the Hidden Self, created to manipulate relationships to meet the Hidden Self's needs (Hillman, 1975).

Precautions: Shadow Work & Trauma

Engaging in shadow work can be a profound and transformative journey, especially for those who have experienced trauma. Handling this process with a Trauma-informed lens is crucial to avoid retraumatization. Navigating the depths of your psyche, confronting hidden aspects of yourself, and integrating these parts into your conscious awareness requires careful preparation and, for those facilitating, proper training. To ensure this process is both safe and effective, it's essential to approach it with care, mindfulness, and a deep reverence for boundaries.

Here are some detailed precautions and steps to guide both facilitators and experiencers to support using shadow work safely and ethically.

Steps for Practitioners

1. **Understand the Limits of Your Expertise**: Recognize the boundaries of your training. If you are not a licensed therapist, be aware of the complexity of trauma and its potential to cause harm if not handled correctly. Know when to refer participants to a qualified mental health professional (van der Kolk, 2014; Siegel, 2010a).

2. **Educate Yourself on Trauma**: Learn about trauma—its effects, symptoms, and triggers. Understand concepts such as the window of tolerance, dissociation, and re-traumatization to better recognize signs of distress (Levine, 2015; Ogden et al., 2006).

3. **Consultation**: Engage with Trauma-informed professionals who can offer guidance or supervision. Consider regular consultations to review practices and discuss challenges (Herman, 1992).

4. **Create a Safe Environment**: Ensure that the physical and emotional environment is safe and supportive. This includes clear boundaries, a predictable structure, and allowing participants control over their involvement, permitting them to step back if needed (Porges, 2011).

5. **Practice Informed Consent**: Clearly explain the nature of shadow work, potential risks, and benefits. Ensure that participants are fully aware of what the process involves and provide fully informed consent (Courtois and Ford, 2013).

6. **Develop an Emergency Protocol**: Have a plan in place for handling intense emotional reactions or psychological crises. This might include having contact information for local mental health crisis teams or therapists who agree to be available for referrals (Siegel, 2010b; Courtois and Ford, 2013).

7. **Use a Trauma-Informed Approach**: Approach all activities with sensitivity to the presence of trauma. Avoid forceful encouragement to share deeply personal or traumatic content. Allow participants to determine the pace and depth of their engagement. Be aware of how group dynamics and activities may trigger trauma in participants. For example, large breathwork sessions can be destabilizing for some participants (van der Kolk, 2014).

8. **Ongoing Education and Supervision**: Continue to learn about trauma and shadow work through workshops, courses, and literature. Regular supervision or consultation with Trauma-informed professionals is crucial to maintaining a safe practice (Herman, 1992; Levine, 2015).

Steps for Individuals Engaging in Shadow Work

1. **Create a Safe Physical Space**: Choose an environment where you feel secure and at ease. Surround yourself with grounding objects like soft blankets, calming visuals, and soothing scents. Ensure you won't be disturbed during your sessions by setting clear boundaries with others (Levine, 2015; Siegel, 2010a).

2. **Prepare Yourself Emotionally and Mentally**: Before diving into shadow work, prepare yourself emotionally and mentally. Engage in grounding exercises such as deep breathing, meditation, or gentle stretching. Reflect on your current emotional state and be honest with yourself about any recent triggers or stressors. Set a clear intention for your shadow work session, focusing on what you hope to achieve or understand (van der Kolk, 2014).

3. **Know and Respect Your Limits**: It's crucial to know and respect your limits. Be aware of your emotional and mental boundaries, and commit to honoring them throughout your process. If you begin to feel overwhelmed, give yourself permission to take a break or stop for the day. Remember, it's okay to move at your own pace; healing is not a race (Porges, 2011).

4. **Develop a Post-Session Self-Care Plan**: Plan activities that help you decompress and relax after your shadow work session. This might include taking a warm bath, listening to calming music, or spending time in nature. Have comforting items on hand, such as a favorite book, a cozy blanket, or a trusted pet to cuddle with. Make sure to hydrate and nourish your body with healthy food and plenty of water (Courtois and Ford, 2013).

5. **Build a Support Network**: A support network is essential. Identify friends, family members, or support groups who can offer understanding and empathy. Share your journey with someone you trust, explaining the nature of shadow work and why it's

important to you. Have emergency contacts available, such as a therapist or a crisis hotline, should you need professional support (Herman, 1992).

6. **Practice Regular Self-Care**: Through regular self-care, you can build resilience and maintain emotional balance. Engage in activities that bring you joy and fulfillment, whether it's creative pursuits, physical exercise, or quiet reflection. Ensure you get adequate rest and practice good sleep hygiene (Ogden et al., 2006).

7. **Educate Yourself About Shadow Work**: Read books, articles, and other resources to deepen your understanding of shadow work and its potential impacts. Learn about different techniques and approaches, and decide which ones resonate most with you. Stay informed about how trauma can manifest and affect your shadow work journey (Jung, 1969b; Levine, 2015).

8. **Stay Grounded and Present**: During sessions, grounding techniques are vital. Use grounding exercises to help maintain stability throughout your session. Focus on your breath, feel your feet on the ground, or hold a grounding object. If you start to feel detached or dissociated, gently bring your awareness back to the present moment by naming objects in the room or describing their colors and textures (Scott-Alexander, 2023). Remind yourself that you are safe and in control of your process (Siegel, 2010a).

9. **Listen to Your Inner Wisdom**: Pay close attention to your body's signals and emotional cues. If something feels too intense or uncomfortable, respect that feeling and take a step back. Use journaling as a tool to process your thoughts and emotions, capturing any insights or realizations that emerge. Trust your intuition and inner guidance as you navigate your shadow work journey (Jung, 1969a).

10. **Integrate Your Experiences**: Integration is a key part of the shadow work process. After each session, take time to reflect on what you've discovered and how it relates to your overall journey. Find ways to integrate these insights into your daily life, whether through changes in behavior, new coping strategies, or shifts in

perspective. Celebrate your progress, no matter how small, and acknowledge the courage it takes to confront and embrace your shadow (Levine, 2015; Ogden et al., 2006).

11. **Tap into Healing Energies**: Tap into the healing energy you experienced during your non-ordinary state encounters. Whether it was an inner presence, an external guide, or the spirit of plant medicine, invite this energy to support you during your shadow work. Visualize this energy surrounding and protecting you, offering guidance and comfort as you navigate your inner landscape. Stay open to any messages or insights that may come from this connection and use them to bolster your resolve and sense of safety (Siegel, 2010b).

12. **Regularly Check in With Yourself**: This is important to gauge how the shadow work is impacting you. Adjust your approach as needed to ensure you remain grounded and supported. Keep track of your journey through journaling or creating art, allowing you to see your growth and development over time (van der Kolk, 2014).

By taking these steps, you can ensure that your engagement in shadow work is conducted with care and respect for your well-being. This mindful approach helps prevent retraumatization and fosters a deeper, more compassionate understanding of yourself, leading to profound healing and integration.

The Trauma Vortex vs the Healing Vortex

In trauma therapy, two important concepts—introduced by Dr. Peter Levine, a trauma expert—are the "healing vortex" and the "trauma vortex" (Levine and Frederick, 1997). These represent the contrasting experiences individuals may face during therapy and the pathways toward recovery. Understanding both vortices helps clients and practitioners navigate the complex terrain of trauma healing.

Trauma Vortex

The trauma vortex embodies the overwhelming emotional and physiological responses often triggered by trauma. When individuals are caught in this vortex, they re-experience the distress of trauma, making it difficult to function in the present moment.

Characteristics

- **Emotional intensity:** Deep feelings of fear, grief, or rage (Levine, 2010).
- **Physical symptoms:** Tension, frozen sensations, or even somatic pain (Ogden et al., 2006).
- **Intrusive memories:** Flashbacks or distressing thoughts connected to the trauma (Rothschild, 2000).
- **Avoidance:** Attempting to sidestep reminders of trauma, leading to isolation (van der Kolk, 2014).
- **Negative self-perception:** Shame, guilt, or feelings of worthlessness (Herman, 1992).

Importance

Understanding the trauma vortex is essential for both practitioners and clients because it helps to identify when trauma is taking control. Recognizing the signs of overwhelm enables the creation of strategies for managing these intense reactions. This understanding helps establish a safe environment for processing trauma and identifying potential triggers (Levine and Frederick, 1997).

Healing Vortex

The healing vortex, in contrast, represents the restorative processes that help individuals move toward recovery. This includes the body's natural healing capacities, fostering a sense of empowerment, and re-establishing emotional and physical safety.

Characteristics

- **Calm and safety:** Feeling grounded and secure within the body and mind (Levine and Frederick, 1997).
- **Emotional regulation:** A growing ability to manage and process emotions (Porges, 2011).
- **Resilience:** Increased capacity to recover from stressful experiences (Siegel, 2012b).

- **Positive connections:** Building stronger, supportive relationships (van der Kolk, 2014).
- **Empowerment:** Developing self-agency and confidence in handling life's challenges (Herman, 1992).

Importance

In trauma therapy, fostering the healing vortex is crucial because it counterbalances the trauma vortex. The goal is to help individuals move from a state of overwhelm to one of resilience and growth. This is achieved by creating safe, supportive experiences that promote healing, empowerment, and connection (Levine and Frederick, 1997).

Integration in Therapy

In Trauma-informed therapy, balancing both the trauma and healing vortices is vital. The practitioner guides clients through navigating both spaces, ensuring that they don't become overwhelmed by trauma while fostering experiences that build resilience (Levine, 2010). Techniques such as grounding, mindfulness, and somatic experiencing support the healing vortex, while trauma processing methods help diminish the intensity of the trauma vortex (Levine and Frederick, 1997).

Before venturing into painful memories or emotions, it's essential to first establish what healing feels like in the body. The healing vortex becomes a safe space to relax into a new way of being. Only then can one safely dip into trauma without being consumed by the intensity of the trauma vortex (Rothschild, 2000).

Above all, working from a person-centered lens is essential. This means tracking and honoring the unique needs of each individual, ensuring that they feel supported in their healing journey (Siegel, 2012).

By understanding and utilizing these concepts, therapists create a balanced approach to help clients move from a state of distress to one of well-being and resilience (Levine, 2010).

Ensuring Safe and Supportive Trauma-Informed Shadow Work
During Sessions

- **Grounding Techniques**: Equip yourself and participants with grounding techniques to manage emotional distress. Techniques such as deep breathing, body awareness, and sensory focus can establish a foundation of safety and stability during shadow work sessions (Levine, 2010; Porges, 2011). Teaching these techniques at the start of sessions allows participants to maintain presence and reduce dissociation.

- **Monitoring**: Keep an attentive watch for signs of distress, such as dissociation, hyperventilation, or emotional withdrawal. Trauma-informed practitioners should intervene with gentle grounding techniques or offer breaks when necessary to ensure participants remain connected and calm (Herman, 1992; Ogden et al., 2006). This attunement to the participant's emotional state is critical for preventing re-traumatization.

- **Flexibility**: Modify or halt the process based on the participant's response. Prioritizing the individual's well-being over the session's agenda promotes a safe environment. This adaptability ensures the participant feels in control and supported throughout the session (Rothschild, 2000).

- **Integrate Mindfulness**: Encourage practices that enhance mindfulness and present-moment awareness. Mindfulness practices, such as focusing on breath or body sensations, can help participants stay grounded in the present, preventing overwhelming immersion into traumatic memories (Kabat-Zinn, 1990; van der Kolk, 2014). Fostering mindfulness during shadow work can enhance the participant's ability to navigate emotional content safely.

- **Emphasize Personal Agency**: Reinforce the participant's personal agency by encouraging them to make decisions about their healing journey. This empowerment can help counteract the feelings of helplessness often associated with trauma (Herman, 1992; Levine and Frederick, 1997). Allowing participants to set their own pace fosters autonomy and strengthens resilience.

- **Gradual Exposure**: Avoid deep diving into traumatic memories abruptly. Gradual exposure to difficult content builds trust and helps participants develop the capacity to confront deeper psychological material (Ogden et al., 2006). This process prevents overwhelm and supports the integration of insights at a manageable pace.

Post–Session

- **Debriefing**: Allocate time after each session for participants to reflect on and discuss their experiences in a supportive environment. Debriefing helps to consolidate insights gained during the session and promotes emotional integration (Levine and Frederick, 1997). Providing validation and allowing participants to share their experiences encourages a sense of connection and healing.
- **Follow Up**: Offer participants resources for continued support, such as therapist referrals or support groups. Making yourself available for post-session concerns reassures participants that they are not alone in their healing journey (Rothschild, 2000; van der Kolk, 2014).

Conclusion

Facilitating Trauma-informed shadow work requires careful preparation, acute awareness of participants' emotional states, and the ability to adapt or refer to professionals as necessary. By prioritizing safety, flexibility, and personal agency, shadow work can become a transformative process of self-discovery and healing, rather than a potential source of retraumatization (Levine, 2010; Ogden et al., 2006). Through the use of grounding, mindfulness, and ongoing support, practitioners can ensure that individuals navigating shadow work feel both confident and cared for as they explore their inner landscapes.

The Effectiveness of Black Paper in Art Therapy

As an Art Therapist, I always have black paper on hand for clients with materials that will show up vividly like metallic paint, metallic pens, puffy paint, acrylic markers, and chalk (soft) pastels. The use of black paper in Art Therapy offers a profound medium that can evoke, process, and transform various emotional states. Here's how it facilitates the therapeutic process in several significant ways, supported by Art Therapy theory and practice:

1. **Healing from Depression**: Black paper allows for the creation of highlights rather than shadows, symbolically shifting focus from darkness to light. This mirrors therapeutic goals in depression treatment, where the process of creation on a dark background

can help clients shift their internal perspective toward hope and light. Research on Art Therapy for depression highlights the power of symbols and metaphor in shifting clients' cognitive and emotional patterns.

2. **Shadow Work**: Black paper is a fitting medium for "shadow work" as it connects with Jungian concepts of the unconscious. The black background can represent the shadow aspects of self, allowing these aspects to be symbolically expanded upon and integrated. According to Jungian psychology, engaging with the shadow can lead to profound personal transformation (Jung, 1979).

3. **Contrast and Visibility**: Using light-colored or metallic mediums on black paper emphasizes contrast, bringing the artwork to life in ways that differ from working on a white canvas. This increased visibility of the artwork's details may help clients see their emotional expressions more clearly, supporting the therapeutic process of self-reflection and insight (Case and Dalley, 2014).

4. **Expression of Emotions**: Black paper evokes deeper, often repressed emotions like grief, sadness, or fear. The darkness of the paper can serve as a non-verbal expression of these feelings, particularly useful for clients who struggle with verbal communication. Art Therapists emphasize that non-verbal expression in Art Therapy can help access and process emotions that are otherwise difficult to articulate (McNiff, 2004).

5. **Focus and Attention**: Working on black paper requires a shift in cognitive processes, where the artist focuses on creating light rather than shading darkness. This reversal can stimulate different parts of the brain and encourage creativity, fostering cognitive flexibility, problem-solving, and the development of new perspectives, crucial for emotional healing (Ganim and Fox, 1999).

6. **Reduction of Stimuli**: For some clients, the brightness of a white page can be overwhelming. Black paper reduces this visual intensity and may feel less stimulating, creating a more soothing starting point for individuals who experience sensory overload or anxiety.

7. **Highlighting Specific Art Media**: Materials like metallic pens, chalk pastels, and fluorescent colors stand out on black paper,

allowing for specific elements of the artwork to be highlighted. This can be used in therapy to draw attention to significant emotional or symbolic elements in the client's work, facilitating deeper discussion and insight (Moon, 2002b).

8. **Symbolic Meanings**: Black carries rich symbolic meanings across cultures, often representing the unconscious, mystery, and potential. Utilizing black paper taps into these symbolic layers, adding depth to the therapeutic process as clients explore aspects of the unknown or suppressed parts of their psyche (Jung, 1959).

9. **Encouraging Creativity**: Black paper as a non-traditional medium encourages clients to think outside the box and experiment with different materials. This can be particularly freeing for clients who feel constrained by more conventional artistic methods, fostering greater emotional expression and problem-solving (Rubin, 2001).

The selection of black paper in Art Therapy is more than an aesthetic choice; it serves as a powerful tool for emotional exploration, shadow work, and cognitive shift, while facilitating a safe and supportive environment for processing complex feelings.

Art Directive: Shadow Art

Part One

Materials Needed

- 2 pieces of Black paper (9 × 12 or larger)
- Chalk Pastels/ Oil Pastels/ Acrylic Markers

Directions

In this directive, you are invited to connect with your **Self-energy**—the core of your being that represents safety, wisdom, and love. Remember back to the meditation and art directive in module three where you were invited to connect to an inner resource, that part within you that radiates well-being, described as Self-energy. In this directive, you are invited again to create an image to represent that aspect of yourself on black paper.

Allow yourself to sense a place inside where you feel well-being, where all is well.

1. **Sense and Expand**:
   - Begin by focusing inward, identifying a place of calm and strength within.
   - As you breathe, notice if this space expands or brightens. Can you direct your breath to this area, connecting with your **Inner Healer**?
   - Visualize any colors, textures, or shapes that emerge from this space. This felt sense symbolizes your core energy, where safety and love reside.
2. **Receive Messages:**
   - Ask if this space has any messages for you. Stay open to the insights that come, and express gratitude for this connection.
3. **Create:**
   - After your meditation, begin creating on black paper. Use your art materials to represent the sensations, colors, or images you encountered during your visualization.

This artwork serves as a visual reminder of your **inner strength** and connection to **Self-energy**.

Part Two

In this section, you're invited to explore a different aspect of the self—your **shadow**. I've developed and refined this directive over the years to support both my clients and my own personal growth. The language used throughout this directive is influenced by the Internal Family Systems (IFS) approach. Using a piece of black paper (or the same one if you prefer), create images that represent parts of yourself that you may not fully embrace.

This can be a part of you that:

- **You don't like.**
- **You feel shame over.**
- **You wish to change.**

Alternatively, allow your unconscious mind to guide the process, letting images emerge organically as you connect with these hidden parts of your psyche.

1. **Process:**
   - Stay grounded, keeping in mind the first directive you created, which represents your strengths.
   - Breathe deeply as you work through this process, feeling your connection to Self-energy.

2. **Reflection:**
   - Once your shadow piece is complete, take some time to look at your image and engage with it.
   - Is there anything it needs to say? A message for you?
   - Ask if it knows how old you currently are.
   - Be curious. When did it first develop in your system? It would have developed when you needed it and when Self-energy was not present.
   - Acknowledge it for the work it has been doing and the role this part has played in your life.
   - Is it aware that you currently have Self-energy? It may not know this and may not even trust this as it was born at a time when there was none. This process of building trust can take time. That is ok.
   - Ask if it would like to take a rest and do what it would rather be doing. Let it know that your Self-energy can support it in doing that. It doesn't need to work so hard anymore.

3. **Journal:**
   - Reflect on the insights that emerged during this process. Journal about the relationship between your Self-energy and shadow aspects, and how this work may have deepened your understanding of yourself.

Art Directive: Welcoming the Unwelcome Parts of Self

Create a 3-D Image of Your Shadow Self & All It Represents

In this directive, we will work toward the integration of our Shadow side. As stated earlier, the more we deny or push away our Shadow side, the darker it gets, and the stronger a hold it begins to have over our lives. By accepting the parts of ourselves that feel uncomfortable, we shed light on them, removing shame as we give them a voice. At the same time, we cultivate deeper compassion as we begin to understand where they came from, why they arose, and their purpose, which is often to protect us.

Materials Needed

- Clay
- Spray bottle with water
- Bowl of water
- Paper towel
- Carving Tools: Popsicle stick, something sharp for creating details if needed (could use chopsticks), wire, string, or tooth floss for cutting clay if needed
- A paper plate or a movable hard surface to create your image on and allow it to dry
- Plastic Wrap (optional)
- Resource Image from Module 3

To Begin

Start by connecting with your breath and noticing any sensations or feelings in the body. Observe any new areas of tension. Working with our Shadow can sometimes bring up new and uncomfortable feelings. Know that whatever is inside you is in divine perfection and not to be feared.

Through this work, we will develop an awareness and acceptance of the other side of our light. Within everything is light and darkness; you can't have a shadow without light casting it. We will work to lighten the darkness by acknowledging it.

As you continue connecting to your breath and body, notice if there is a part within you that feels alien, separate, or even unacceptable. Breathe into the space this feeling occupies within you, wherever it may be. Stay with your breath and feel your body rooted to the ground, supported. Know that you are loved, and it is safe to explore these parts of yourself.

If at any moment you feel unsafe, bring out the resource image you created in Module 3 and keep it near, imagining a cocoon of light surrounding and protecting you. Maybe even call in your guardian spirits, angels, or whatever higher power you resonate with. Know that you are safe and protected and nothing will come up that you are not yet ready to move.

If at any point you feel like stopping, remember that you are in control of this process. Stay connected to your breath, inhaling through the nose, expanding the belly, lungs, and side ribs for a full, complete breath before slowly exhaling through the mouth, feeling a deeper connection to the earth with every exhale and a release of any fears, stresses, or uncomfortable feelings.

1. **Identify Your Shadow**: Focus on the part of yourself that feels alien, separate, or uncomfortable. See if there is an image, color, or sensation that could embody or personify this feeling within. Something that would help you identify it more clearly.

2. **Felt Sense**: Once you have this image in mind, notice the felt sense it evokes in you. Is it prickly, jumpy, agitated, smooth, wet? Whatever comes up for you is the right answer.

3. **Give it Space:** Now that you have identified a felt sense and an image, feel yourself being with this part of yourself, possibly even sitting next to it with a sense of wonder, compassion, and curiosity. Be aware not to judge it but just be with it in an accepting manner. Nothing needs to be said or communicated at this point; you are just giving this part of yourself space to be. Notice if the felt sense of your image, object, or sensation changes as you sit with it.

4. **Dialogue with the Shadow**: Ask this part of yourself if it has anything it would like to say or a message it would like to give you. Wait in a comfortable, receptive manner to see what words or messages may rise from your shadow. If nothing comes up, see if there is a color, shape, or another sensation it has that would feel appropriate as an expression of itself.

5. **Acknowledgment**: Thank your Shadow for this information and for showing itself to you. Especially if your Shadow is used to hiding, this can be a significant step in its integration.

6. **Shape the Clay**: When you feel your dialogue is complete, stay connected to your inner sensations and come back into the room. You may even keep your eyes closed. Now grab your piece of clay.

Ensure it is soft and malleable. Plasticine or play-doh can also be used, though the smell and texture of real earth clay will be the most grounding.

7. **Working Somatically:** Begin moving your hands through the clay, fully feeling the temperature, smell, and sensation between each finger and your palms. Stay connected to your breath.

8. **Trust the Process:** Allow a shape to emerge, knowing it already exists within the clay. Move the clay to uncover what is lying underneath, hiding. Allow your Shadow to be expressed in 3-D form. Continue working with your depiction until it feels complete. Use a spray bottle and a bowl of water to wet the clay as needed. Water is an excellent conduit for releasing emotions.

9. **Release Shame:** This part of you may not have often shown itself, and when it has, there may have been a deep sense of shame. You are allowing it to be revealed, knowing it holds beauty, value, and worth. Your Shadow has supported you in the only way it knew, and now it is time to reveal it. Stay curious as its form emerges and changes while you remove the layers hiding it. Speak to it tenderly as you remove these layers, letting it know it is safe to show itself.

10. **Reflection:** This process can take a long time, so only stop when it feels right. Stay connected to your breath, mindful of your feet on the ground or your seat touching the chair. Once you feel complete, look at what you have created. Spend some time with it. Notice any feelings that come up and keep your journal close to write down any messages or insights.

11. **What Does It Need:** As you sit with your Shadow, see if there are any other messages it has for you. Ask what it has always wanted to say, where it came from, what created it, and what it needs to feel safe and loved. Is there anything you can give it that it needs at this moment? Let it know that it no longer needs to work so hard and ask what it would rather be doing. Offer your Shadow part some of your own Self-energy, sharing with it that this energy that you now possess can help it heal and be seen.

12. **Integration:** Remember, this part of you may feel unwanted and unloved. You may not want this part of you anymore. But before letting it go, closure and acceptance of the ways your Shadow

has helped you can assist in its integration. Notice how it has protected you, even in ways that seemed unnecessary, unconventional, or unhelpful. As mentioned before, these parts often develop at a young age and express themselves in childlike ways. Thank your Shadow for its service before releasing it from the dark confines of your psyche.

13. **Releasing and Transmuting:** If you are saying goodbye to your Shadow, is there anything you need to fill the area it occupied? Breathe into this space and notice any sensations. Call in your guides if needed or look to your resource image for support.

14. **Closure**: Envision the changes in your life with this part of yourself now integrated and no longer having a strong unconscious hold over you. Write these in your journal and allow some time for quiet reflection, letting all revelations come to the surface.

15. **Reflections**: By working with the Shadow in a tangible, 3-D form, we are bringing the unconscious into consciousness, a powerful step toward healing and self-awareness. This process, like all shadow work, is not always easy, but it holds the potential for deep transformation and compassion for the parts of ourselves we may have hidden away for years.

Meditation: Healing Addictive Patterns

Posture

Sit comfortably in Easy Pose with your legs crossed. Gently tuck your neck to lengthen the upper spine, a technique often called neck lock or Jalandhar bandh. Sit up straight, feeling grounded and connected to the earth beneath you.

Hand Mudra

Form fists with both hands, extending your thumbs out straight. Place your thumbs on your temples, finding the natural niche where they fit. Apply firm pressure with your fists facing forward.

- Additional Detail: Clench your back molars and keep your lips closed. Squeeze the molars tightly and then release, feeling the muscle rhythmically move under your thumbs. This motion will massage your thumbs as you maintain firm pressure with your hands.

Eyes

Close your eyes and focus on the area of the forehead in between the eye brows, sometimes referred to as the **Third Eye**.

Mantra

Silently chant the five primal sounds, known as the Panj Shabd: **Sa-Ta-Na-Ma**, which symbolize birth, life, death, and rebirth. Keep your focus on the brow point or third eye, as you recite the mantra. (The fifth sound represented is **Aa** – embodying the **totality** or **oneness** with the universe, which is not chanted alone but included in these four listed).

Time

Practice this meditation for 5–31 minutes.

Explanation

This meditation targets the central area of the brain, especially beneath the pineal gland. In Yogic science, it's believed that imbalances in this region contribute to persistent mental and physical addictions. This practice aims to stimulate the secretion of neurochemicals from the pineal gland, helping to break free from old patterns and addictive behaviors.

Note on Practice

As already mentioned, many different teachings speak of habitual patterns being formed or broken in 40-day cycles. That's why this book emphasizes maintaining a 40-day meditation routine. More deeply ingrained patterns might take longer to overcome. Addictions can be related to substances like sugar, tobacco, drugs, or alcohol, as well as behaviors like expecting rejection, lack of confidence, insecurity, pessimism, or any persistent pattern that feels inescapable.

By dedicating yourself to this practice, you can begin to shift these patterns and create a path toward greater freedom and self-mastery.

Journaling & Shining Light on Your Shadow

Now that you have created an image of what your Shadow looks like, I invite you to write a letter, from your Shadow to yourself. As you write this letter, write it in the first person from their point of view for why they do what they do. This is a part of you but write it to yourself as if this part (Shadow) were disconnected from you. Feel all the emotions that may come to the surface from your Shadow part. These emotions need to be released and although it may be uncomfortable for some, the rise of these emotions is what assists in the release. Allow them to flow. If you feel like answering your Shadow as you write, take the time to do this either verbally or in written form.

1. **Communicate with Your Shadow:** Ask your Shadow part what it would rather be doing if it wasn't working so hard all these years. Would it rather be doing that now instead? Let your Shadow part know that it no longer needs to work so hard, that you are here to listen to it and allow light to shine on it. Ask your Shadow part how old it thinks you are. Let it know your actual age, let it know that you now have the tools and strength to support yourself and it no longer needs to work so hard. Give it permission to take a break, to rest. Create trust with your shadow, as you feel into your own inner strength and sense of self, letting it know you are in charge and can support yourself. This is a very powerful moment within this exercise. Breathe.

2. **Reflect and Adjust:** Once you have finished writing this letter, look at your artwork and check in if there are any changes in this physical representation of your Shadow needs. Often, after we have released some of the pressure that our Shadow side holds, we require a shift in how we have represented it. This will help in the healing that is taking place. You are creating not only a new relationship with this part of you that has been hidden (or in the shadows), but you are also creating a new version of a part of you whose ways of coping in the world may no longer be serving you. Breathe deeply into this experience and feel it being grounded into the earth for it to transmute, change, and be reborn.

Dreamwork: Understanding the Patterns

Throughout the modules in this book, you have been invited to record and keep track of your dreams, creating art and journaling to further decipher what deeper meanings they have held.

Now we will take this one step further to look for patterns or themes that have been quietly whispering to us; an inner truth we may have been unaware of.

1. **Finding a Quiet Place:** After your yoga, meditation, or a nice bath, find a quiet place where you will not be interrupted and begin to read through your dream journal and look at the artwork you made.

2. **Identifying Patterns:** Are there words, phrases, colors, or images that are repeated? On a separate page, begin writing these out. It may be helpful to use a large piece of paper and a marker to begin mapping what patterns you recognize. Are there people that continue to show up? Situations? How do you show up in the dream? Are there consistencies in this? Create a map or a diagram labeling the themes that you see. Using different colors to identify themes can be helpful.

3. **Clustering Themes:** Once you have identified themes, begin clustering these into their own categories. Stay open to any information or intuitive sensations that come up as you continue through this process, even writing messages down as they pop into your head. We are looking for the underlying meaning and overall themes within your life. These can have both positive and negative associations; all are good and have meaning.

4. **Reflecting on Origins:** Once you have identified themes and clustered these into their own categories, imagine where these may have developed in your life. Knowing that the current lens we look through to see the world is always clouded by past experiences, ask yourself if your lens has been clouded and how it got that way. Is there anything that needs to come to the surface to be moved from the psyche, to be cleared and cleaned? This is your process, so stay open to what you may need at this moment, keeping an open and curious acceptance of whatever arises.

5. **Taking Inventory:** Take inventory of the growth that you may see from when you first began this book. Look for that, and it will be revealed. It is when we can take inventory of how much we have grown and healed that we can really begin to feel an internal shift of change within the mind and body.

Often it is within our dreams that our Shadow-self emerges. Do you notice any shadow aspects of you within the themes and patterns? If so, what is your Shadow-self needing to say?

How Are You Doing with Your 40-Day Practice?

As we move into the seventh module of this program, your daily practice is more important than ever. This module dives the deepest into our psyche. Supporting yourself through this process is pivotal in creating lasting healing.

How has your daily meditation practice been supporting you so far? Have you continued with the original meditation, or have you found another that you enjoy? Maybe you are moving forward with a 90, 120, or even 1000-day meditation practice?

Where do you usually practice your daily meditation? Establishing a consistent sacred space for meditation helps to cultivate an energy field that deepens your practice over time. This space becomes a sanctuary, allowing you to drop more quickly into theta brainwave states or deeper meditative experiences (Davidson and Lutz, 2008).

Are there any tokens or talismans you would like to include in your space as a reminder of the etheric support in your life? Perhaps you could include crystals, photos of loved ones, or even a picture of yourself as a child. Surrounding yourself with these peaceful supports can bring comfort and grounding as you continue your journey into regular meditation practice. Don't forget to journal afterward, so you can reflect on your progress and insights over time (Siegel, 2012).

SUMMARY: Integrating Our Shadow Side

This module focuses on the integration of the shadow side within the context of psychedelic experiences, emphasizing the importance of bringing unconscious aspects of the self into conscious awareness for healing and growth. Psychedelics can be powerful tools in revealing hidden parts of the psyche, making this work particularly relevant for those using these substances for personal transformation. This process involves acknowledging and integrating these shadow parts to lessen their hold on us. When left unaddressed, these parts can manifest as insecurities, judgments, self-loathing, and other negative traits that hinder our highest expression of self. The module emphasizes accepting these less desirable parts as integral to our being.

Key Support Elements for Your Journey:

1. **Getting to Know and Love Your Shadow:**
   This section introduces the shadow concept and its relevance to psychedelic integration. Psychedelics often bring buried aspects of the Self to the surface, providing a unique opportunity to acknowledge, confront, and integrate these shadow parts. By learning to accept and work with the Shadow, individuals can dissolve its intensity, allowing for a more authentic and holistic self-expression.

2. **Jungian Psychology:**
   Carl Jung's teachings on the Shadow are explored in this section, providing a framework for understanding the unconscious material that Psychedelics can unearth. The module emphasizes that by integrating these shadow aspects, individuals can achieve a more balanced and whole sense of Self, which is a critical goal in the integration process following psychedelic experiences.

3. **Precautions: Shadow Work & Trauma:**
   Given the powerful and sometimes overwhelming nature of psychedelic experiences, this section highlights the importance of a Trauma-informed approach to shadow work. It provides practical steps to ensure that the process is conducted safely, avoiding retraumatization, which can be a risk when deep, unconscious material surfaces during or after a psychedelic journey.

4. **The Trauma Vortex vs the Healing Vortex:**
   This section introduces the concepts of the trauma vortex and the healing vortex, which are particularly relevant in the aftermath of intense psychedelic experiences. Understanding these

concepts helps one navigate the integration process by balancing the potentially destabilizing effects of trauma with the restorative aspects of healing that Psychedelics can facilitate.

5. **Ensuring Safe and Supportive Trauma-Informed Shadow Work:**

    This section provides guidelines for creating a safe environment during Shadow work, which is essential for effectively integrating the insights gained from Psychedelics. It emphasizes grounding techniques, mindfulness, and maintaining personal agency to support individuals in processing the deep material that may arise during or after psychedelic sessions.

6. **The Effectiveness of Black Paper in Art Therapy:**

    Black paper is used as a tool in Art Therapy to explore and express the deep, often dark emotions that Psychedelics can bring to the surface. This section discusses how using black paper can help individuals visually process and integrate these emotions, making it a powerful method for those working with psychedelic experiences.

7. **Art Directive: Shadow Art:**

    This art directive involves creating visual representations of inner resources and Shadow aspects, which can be directly connected to the images and emotions experienced during a psychedelic journey. This exercise supports the integration process by helping to externalize and better understand the Shadow material brought up by Psychedelics.

8. **Art Directive: Welcoming the Unwelcome Parts of Self:**

    This directive invites you to create a 3-D image of your Shadow-self, facilitating the integration of difficult or unwelcome aspects of the psyche that Psychedelics may reveal. By physically manifesting these parts in art, you can begin to accept and transform them, which is a crucial step in the integration process.

9. **Meditation: Healing Addictive Patterns:**

    The meditation introduced here focuses on breaking free from addictive patterns, a common issue that Psychedelics often bring to light. This practice supports the integration process by helping one shift away from old habits and behaviors that may have surfaced during psychedelic experiences, fostering greater freedom and self-mastery.

10. **Journaling & Shining Light on Your Shadow:**

   Journaling is used as a tool to communicate with and understand the Shadow-self, which Psychedelics can vividly expose. This exercise allows for the processing and integration of the emotions and insights from your psychedelic experience, promoting a deeper understanding of the shadow's role in your life.

11. **Dreamwork: Understanding the Patterns:**

   In this chapter of dreamwork, you are invited to analyze your dreams to find any recurring patterns related to your Shadow parts, which may have been highlighted or triggered by your psychedelic experience. Understanding these patterns is essential for integrating the Shadow aspects revealed by Psychedelics, leading to a more unified and conscious self.

Throughout this module, you are guided to approach your shadow with compassion and curiosity, using a variety of therapeutic tools and practices to integrate these aspects into your life. When using Psychedelics for healing, this work is especially important, as it helps to process and make sense of the profound, often challenging material that these substances can bring to the forefront of consciousness.

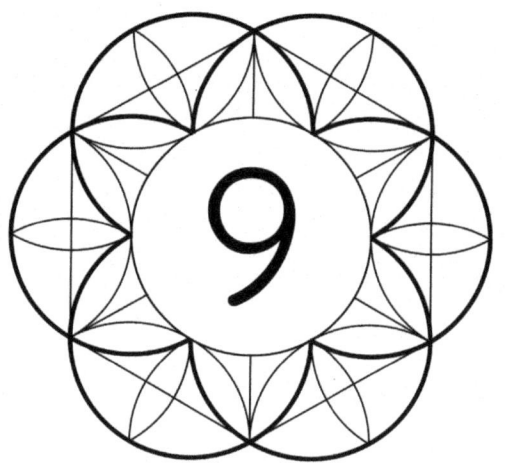

MODULE 9
CHOOSE YOUR LIFE

Psychedelic Integration: Embracing Your New Path

The psychedelic experience may have opened a path toward a new life filled with growth and healing, but it is you who has continued the journey in forging that path. Celebrate yourself for the work you have done and embrace the possibilities that lie ahead from this point onward.

Life can often feel cyclical, with similar issues sometimes arising repeatedly. This may seem defeating when we find ourselves revisiting past feelings or challenges. However, you are now in a different place. Consider life as a spiral that ascends upward. Although you may revisit uncomfortable feelings and memories, you now possess tools that allow you to navigate these experiences with greater ease and move through them at a quicker pace than before. You have come this far and have done tremendous work to get here. Celebrate your efforts and recognize that despite hardships, you have cultivated resilience, tenacity, and a deep inner connection to that essential part of yourself—your Soul. Jung (1933) described this process as individuation, where we move towards integrating different aspects of the self, including shadow elements, in order to achieve greater wholeness.

Many believe that this journey of self-connection and Soul-discovery is the purpose of life (Jung, 1966). This deep connection can provide strength, compassion, and an inner drive toward living life fully and presently. As you embody this new way of being, the positive effects reverberate into all living things because we are interconnected. When you heal, your journey touches the lives of those around you. At times, this may lead to others moving away from your path, which can be difficult, but it is crucial to ensure that you are filling your own cup first, so that what you give to the world comes from an overflow of what you have nurtured within yourself (Harris, 2019b).

Now that your slate has been washed clean through your psychedelic experience and the integration work you've done, it's time to focus on creating and choosing the life you want to live. The time is now to embrace the new you and stand strong and proud of who you are. Focusing on the gifts and tools cultivated through your experience, you are invited to manifest a life that is in perfect alignment with your Soul's path (Carhart-Harris and Friston, 2019).

Visualize Your Ideal Life

What do you want your life to look like? Take time to journal about this throughout the module, allowing any thoughts that arise to be written down.

Turn Inward

Continue the practice of turning inward through meditation, artistic reflection, and journaling for deeper awareness. These practices can empower you to see the world in a new way, one of your own choosing.

Choose Your Life: Questions Needing Answers

Now that you have moved through the first eight modules of this book, we arrive at a place of choice grounded in your healing experience. Let's begin with a few questions:

- What do you want in your life?
- What do you need to sustain your healing and growth?
- How will you go about bringing that to fruition?

Keep these questions in mind as we move through this module. Write them in your journal and begin brainstorming answers that feel true to you. Your non-ordinary state has opened the doors of perception, so be open to whatever information comes to you (Carhart-Harris and Friston, 2019).

Making Choices to Support Your New Life

I invite you to write out a list of what your life was like before starting this journey. Note the pieces that felt supportive and those that did not. Consider the parts that continued to surface despite being rooted in the past—elements that may have held you back or even debilitated you (Jung, 1966). Also, reflect on the changes you have felt since embarking on this journey of self-discovery toward living your best life.

This process may bring up strong emotions, so before you begin, ensure that you have created a nurturing environment. This space should allow you to work uninterrupted, surrounded by objects that help you feel connected to yourself and to any supportive energies around you (Grof, 2008b).

This exercise is most beneficial after meditation, particularly one that connects you to your inner self and strengths. You might consider using different colored pens to describe various internal experiences or events that have occurred along your journey.

To Begin

1. **Reflect on Relationships**: As you continue to reflect, ask yourself what your relationship is now to:
   - Spirit
   - Self
   - The World

   Note any insights that arise to support you in strengthening these relationships. Reflect on how these relationships have evolved since your psychedelic experience and since engaging with this book (Grof and Halifax, 1977).

2. **Future Visioning:**
   - What would you like these relationships to look like in one month?
   - Six months?
   - One year?

- Five years?

Reflect on how your connection to these relationships will shape your future. Take the time to fully feel these reflections (Siegel, 2012).

3. **Visualization:**
   - Imagine yourself in the future, in relationship with Spirit, Self, and the World. What does your life look like? What do you look like? What are you wearing? What are you doing? How do you spend your days? What fulfills your heart in this future image? Spend time in this reflection to get a complete sense of what you are envisioning.

4. **Journaling:**
   - Once you've completed your visualization, begin journaling about the experience. As you write, imagine that you are bringing this future into your present reality. Remember that time is not linear; experience this memory of the future as if it were happening now. Breathe deeply, stay grounded in the present, and feel your feet connected to the earth. Ground this vision of your future (Harris, 2019b).

5. **Creating Your Future:**
   - Is there anything else you would like to add to this memory? Imagine yourself actively creating this future life. You are the creator of your reality—take time to connect with the feeling of control and agency over your own life (Carhart-Harris and Friston, 2019).

Art Directive: My Life as a Fairy Tale

What Has Been Overcome

For lasting change to take effect in our lives, it is essential to periodically take inventory of how far we have come, the obstacles that have been worked through, and how we've managed to overcome them. This art directive will explore your personal journey through the lens of fairy tales and storytelling. It's your story, and you can craft it however you like, with whichever characters you choose. Now, you have the choice of different outcomes and are invited to be creative in how you envision your future.

When working with fairy tales and storytelling, we are engaging with metaphor, which is a powerful tool to shift the reality we live in (Lakoff and Johnson, 1980). Metaphors can help us express complex emotions and situations in ways that the conscious mind often struggles with. Let the metaphors come from the unconscious and be guided by the wisdom of your heart. If you find yourself thinking too hard, gently reconnect to your breath, press your feet into the ground, and allow your intuition to guide you from a creative space.

As you create, be open to the direction that this activity may take. Stay present with how the story evolves and create that in front of you. This can be done on one large piece of paper as a snapshot of your story, or it may take shape across several sheets, representing a beginning, middle, and end. Watch as your story comes to life and be aware of any opportunities for the story to shift and reflect those changes (McNiff, 1992).

To Begin: Your Life in a Fairy Tale

1. What character are you?
2. What is the situation that you must go through or overcome?
3. Who are the supporting characters?
4. Who is the villain?
5. How do you overcome the current situation?
6. What tools does your character use?
7. Is magic used in this fairy tale?
8. What gives your character a sense of empowerment?
9. Use paint, drawing, free art, clay, or other materials to create your story.
10. Write out your story in your journal once finished, noting any changes you may wish to make.

This is a story—pay attention to how outcomes can shift in this format toward positivity. Despite the struggles your character faces, they come out victorious, and every trial provides the strength to overcome adversity. This is the magic of fairy tales. What does your life look like as a fairy tale?

In my early training of Art Therapy, I was fortunate to be a student of Monica Carpendale, Professor Emeritus, and founder of The

Kutenai Art Therapy Institute. She emphasized how studying the metaphors in fairy tales supported a deeper understanding of the trials, tribulations, and collective experiences we go through in life. Through these insights, we can best serve ourselves and our clients when we translate these experiences into art using the lens of the story (Carpendale, 2009).

Meditation for Manifesting Your Future

Begin by quieting the mind and letting go of distractions and attachments. When the mind is focused and clear, its potential for creativity is boundless. Tap into this creative power by practicing directed meditation. Sit comfortably and focus inward, projecting your intentions for the future and your place in the world. For optimal results, practice this meditation on an empty stomach, consuming only liquids throughout the day.

Instructions:

> **Posture:** Sit comfortably with a straight spine.
> **Eye Focus:** Close your eyes.
> **Hand Position/Mudra:** Rest your hands on your knees with palms facing up in Gyan Mudra.

Part One:

1. Take a deep breath in through a rounded mouth with pursed lips and exhale slowly through the nose.
2. Repeat this breathing pattern for 7–15 minutes.

Part Two:

1. Inhale deeply and hold your breath comfortably.
2. Focus on the concept of zero, recognizing that all things are transient and impermanent.
3. Mentally reduce each negative thought and difficult emotion to zero with a single held breath, envisioning them as small points of light fading away.
4. Exhale and repeat, maintaining a steady breathing rhythm.

5. Allow space and time for each negative thought to separately to rise to the surface and consciously imagine that fading to nothing.
6. Continue for 7–11 minutes.

Part Three:

1. Identify a single word representing the quality or condition you desire most for your happiness and growth.
2. Focus on this word, visualizing its various aspects and implications.
3. Inhale deeply and hold your breath as you project this word into the universe with intention.
4. Relax the breath as needed and continue to focus on your chosen word for 5–15 minutes.

To Conclude:

1. Inhale deeply and gently move your shoulders, arms, and spine.
2. Stretch your arms upward, spread your fingers wide, and take a few deep breaths to conclude the meditation session.

Journaling and Reflections

Channeling Your Higher Self

Earlier in this book, you were introduced to a journaling technique that allowed you to access inner wisdom by using different colored pens to ask and answer questions. Now, I invite you to take this practice a step further.

Meditation and Connection

Begin by taking some time in meditation to connect with your Higher Self. This is the aspect of you that is beyond the physical form, the part that holds all the answers and gently guides you on your path. As you meditate, visualize this energy surrounding and filling you, noticing the deep sense of gratitude for this profound connection. The Higher Self, often associated with intuition and spiritual wisdom, has been described as the "True Self" that transcends the ego and is linked to a sense of universal consciousness (Wilber, 2001).

Automatic Writing

From this connected place, engage in automatic writing. This technique involves allowing your hand to move the pen freely, without conscious control, trusting the wisdom that emerges from your inner self (LaChance, 2012). You may begin by asking questions and allowing the answers to flow onto the page, or you can simply start writing continuously, letting the words pour out without overthinking or self-editing.

Spirit of the Medicine

You may also feel called to connect with the spirit of the medicine you used. The essence of this medicine, which now lives within you, can be a source of wisdom and guidance. Psychedelics, when used in a ceremonial or therapeutic context, have often been viewed as vehicles for accessing spiritual or higher consciousness (Grof, 1980). Tap into this energy as a resource for strength and support as you navigate your path. Feel the presence of an etheric team guiding you through the transformative process you are experiencing.

Playing with Colors

As you write, feel the different colors of pens available to you. Let your intuition guide you in choosing which color feels right at the moment, representing different aspects of your inquiry or reflections. Allow yourself to stay open to the process, releasing judgment, and approaching the activity with curiosity and an open heart. This technique supports the process of integrating the emotional and intuitive mind with the logical mind, creating a holistic approach to personal reflection and growth (McNiff, 1992).

Dreamwork

As you complete this program, reflecting on your dream journal can be a helpful way to observe your journey—from where you were before starting, to where you are now. Your psyche has been accompanying you on this path, processing the benefits and healing while you sleep, which has become integrated into who you are today. The connection between dreams and psychological growth is well-documented, as dreams serve as a means for our unconscious mind to process daily events and unresolved emotions (Jung, 1974; Domhoff, 2003).

Reflecting on Your Future Dreams

Reflect now on what dreams you may hold for your future. Imagine your dream state as an ally, working on your behalf while your body rests. The unconscious mind is often thought to play a significant role in personal growth, offering symbolic insights that may not be accessible during waking life (Freud, 1900; Jung, 1974). Before going to bed, set an intention for your dreams to guide you in a way that continues your growth and healing. This aligns with the concept of lucid dreaming and dream incubation, where conscious intentions can influence the content and outcomes of dreams (LaBerge and Rheingold, 1990).

Pay attention to the ideas that surface upon waking and record them. As you practice dream recall and interpretation, you can gain a deeper awareness of unconscious elements in your life that may still require attention or that are evolving (Hartmann, 1998). By making dream journaling a regular practice, you will also strengthen the connection between your conscious mind and your dream world, facilitating greater control and understanding of your inner life.

Dream Decoding

Continue to use the processes discussed in this program to decode your dreams, uncovering deeper insights and awareness. This practice, commonly linked to analytical psychology, allows individuals to derive meaning from dream symbols that represent various parts of the self or unresolved aspects of personal experience (Jung, 1974). Through this decoding, you are empowered to apply those insights in your waking life, enhancing your self-awareness and personal growth.

You are the master of this maze called life, with all its ups and downs. Have faith that whatever life gives you, you now have the tools and resources—stemming from within you—to support your continued journey in creating the life you desire (Siegel, 2012).

Continuing Your 40-Day Practice

You have made it to the final module of this book and have spent time integrating your routine of a 40-day practice into your daily life. Reflect on how this consistency has impacted you. Is there anything you would like to enhance or add to this practice as you continue? How does it feel simply to sit in your meditation space now? Research shows that creating consistent rituals or spaces for mindfulness and meditation can profoundly influence emotional well-being, as our brains begin to associate the environment with calm and centeredness (Siegel, 2012; Davidson et al., 2003).

Do you find that just thinking of your meditation space brings you a sense of peace? Much like memories of challenging experiences can trigger anxiety or stress, positive associations can evoke relaxation and feelings of safety (Levine, 2010).

Have you created an altar or dedicated area within your space that houses items precious to you? This could be an expression of your personal journey—a sacred sanctuary rooted in your healing experience. Notice what emotions come up as you reflect on this space and the time you have spent there. Many find that incorporating tangible items of personal significance into their practice, such as crystals, meaningful photographs, or talismans, can deepen their sense of presence and connection to their spiritual path (Jung, 1974; Kabat-Zinn, 2005).

If this practice has been supportive and grounding, consider making it a continual part of your new life. The benefits of a regular meditation routine—such as enhanced emotional regulation, reduced stress, and increased mindfulness—are cumulative and only deepen over time (Davidson et al., 2003; Kabat-Zinn, 2005). Embrace this practice, and enjoy the ongoing healing and growth it brings to your journey.

Conclusion: Embracing Your Journey Forward

As we come to the close of this transformative journey, I invite you to take a moment to honor and celebrate the profound work you have done. Throughout this program, you have delved deep into the realms of your psyche, explored the hidden corners of your Soul, and bravely faced both light and shadow. This is no small feat. Your commitment to growth, healing, and self-discovery is a testament to your strength and resilience (Jung, 1974; Levine, 2010).

The tools and practices you have learned here are not just for today but are lifelong companions on your path. Meditation, journaling, dreamwork, and artistic expression are doorways to deeper understanding and continuous growth (Kabat-Zinn, 2005; Schore, 2003). They are here for you to return to whenever you need guidance, clarity, or a reminder of your inner strength.

Reflecting on Your Progress

Reflect on the shifts and changes you have experienced since beginning this journey. Think back to where you started and acknowledge how far you have come. The insights gained, the obstacles overcome, and the new perspectives embraced all weave together to form the tapestry of your ongoing transformation (Siegel, 2012).

Take pride in the resiliency you have cultivated. The ability to navigate through life's challenges with greater ease and compassion for yourself is a powerful gift. Remember, every step, no matter how small, is a step forward on this upward spiral path of growth (Davidson et al., 2003).

Continuing the Relationship with Your Inner World

Your inner world is a rich and dynamic landscape that deserves ongoing attention and care. Continue to nurture your relationship with your higher self, the shadow aspects, and all parts of your being. They all hold valuable lessons and wisdom for you (Jung, 1974).

Make time regularly for the practices that resonate with you most. Whether it's sitting in meditation, engaging in creative expression, or reflecting in your journal, these moments of connection will keep you grounded and aligned with your true self (Levine, 2010; Kabat-Zinn, 2005).

Expanding Your Consciousness

The journey of expanding consciousness is endless. There is always more to explore, more to learn, and more ways to grow. Stay curious and open to the new possibilities that life presents. Embrace change as an ally, knowing that with each shift, you are moving closer to your most authentic self (Siegel, 2012).

Set intentions for your continued growth and be open to the guidance that comes from within and from the universe. Trust that you are supported on this path and that the tools you have gained here will serve you well in every phase of your life (Levine, 2010).

Your Role in the World

Remember, your healing and growth ripple out into the world. As you become more attuned to your inner self, you also become a beacon of light and strength for others. Your journey inspires those around you to embark on their own paths of self-discovery and healing (Jung, 1974).

By living authentically and embracing your full self, you contribute to the collective consciousness, fostering a world where everyone can thrive and grow (Kabat-Zinn, 2005).

Summary: Choose Your Life

In this final module, we reflect on the profound journey of growth and healing you have undertaken. While your psychedelic experience may have initiated this new path, it is your continued dedication that has truly shaped and advanced your journey. This module is crafted to help you fully embrace the life path that has emerged from your psychedelic experiences. It aims to solidify the healing and insights you have gained, encouraging you to consciously create and choose the life you wish to live moving forward. Below is an overview of how each section supports the process of psychedelic integration and the intentional creation of your future.

Key Support Elements for Your Journey

1. **Psychedelic Integration: Embracing Your New Path:**
    This section celebrates the work you have done to integrate the lessons and healing from your psychedelic experiences. It encourages you to recognize your resilience and growth, highlighting that the path forward is one of intentional choice. The cyclical nature of life is discussed, with an emphasis on how your newfound tools and insights allow you to navigate recurring challenges with greater ease and awareness.

2. **Choose Your Life: Questions Needing Answers:**
    You are invited to reflect deeply on what you want in your life moving forward. This section poses critical questions to help you define your desires and needs, and how you can bring these into fruition. This reflective process is essential for integrating the clarity and direction gained from psychedelic experiences, ensuring that your choices align with your true self.

3. **Art Directive: My Life as a Fairy Tale:**

   This creative exercise encourages you to view your life as a fairy tale, using metaphor and storytelling to explore your journey. By framing your life in this way, you can better understand the obstacles you've overcome and the strengths you've developed. This process allows you to rewrite your story in a way that empowers you, reflecting the transformative power of Psychedelics and the new narrative you are choosing to live by.

4. **Meditation for Manifesting Your Future:**

   This meditation practice is focused on harnessing the creative potential of your mind to manifest your desired future. It builds on the clarity and intentions formed during psychedelic experiences, helping you project these intentions into the world. The practice emphasizes the importance of focusing inward, clearing distractions, and using directed meditation to create the life you envision.

5. **Journaling and Reflections:**

   In this section, journaling is used as a tool for connecting with your higher self and channeling wisdom gained from your psychedelic journey. The exercise of automatic writing, particularly when connected to the spirit of medicine, allows for deeper insights and guidance as you move forward. This practice supports ongoing integration by keeping you aligned with your inner wisdom and the lessons learned.

6. **Dreamwork:**

   Reflecting on your dreams throughout the processes invited in this book, this section encourages you to continue using dreamwork as a tool for self-understanding and growth. By setting intentions for your dreams and decoding their messages, you can continue to integrate the subconscious material that may have been stirred by your psychedelic experiences. This ongoing practice helps you stay connected to your inner world and the deeper aspects of your psyche.

7. **Conclusion: Embracing Your Journey Forward:**

   The module concludes by inviting you to reflect on the progress you have made and to celebrate the profound work you have done. It encourages you to continue nurturing your relationship with your inner self, using the tools and practices you've learned to guide you through life's challenges. The importance of continuing to expand your consciousness and live authentically is emphasized, as is the ripple effect your healing has on the world around you.

Throughout this module, you are encouraged to take the insights gained from your psychedelic experiences and actively shape your future. As you conclude this transformative journey, honor, and celebrate your achievements. The tools and practices you have learned are lifelong companions on your path. Continue nurturing your relationship with your inner world and stay open to new possibilities. Your healing and growth inspire those around you and contribute to the collective consciousness. Embrace your role in the world, knowing that you are a beacon of light and strength.

Final Thoughts

As we part ways, carry with you the knowledge that you are capable, worthy, and deeply connected to a source of infinite wisdom and love. The journey does not end here; it is ever-evolving. Continue to walk this path with an open heart and a curious mind, knowing that every experience is an opportunity for growth.

You have everything you need within you to create a life filled with joy, purpose, and fulfillment. Embrace the magic of your journey and keep shining your light brightly.

With deep respect and admiration for your courage and commitment,
Charmaine Husum

GLOSSARY

Active Imagination: A journey into the depths of the unconscious mind through imaginative exploration, inviting dialogue with inner figures and visualizations to uncover hidden truths and profound insights. This technique, developed by Carl Jung and exemplified in his work *The Red Book* (published in 2009 but written between 1914 and 1930), allows for profound psychological and spiritual discoveries.

Alan Watts: A British philosopher known for interpreting and popularizing Eastern philosophy for Western audiences. His influential book *The Way of Zen* (1957) explores the principles of Zen Buddhism and its application in daily life.

Alex & Allison Grey: Visionary artists whose work explores the intersection of art, consciousness, and spirituality. Their intricate paintings, such as those in Alex Grey's *Sacred Mirrors* (1990), offer profound insights into the human experience and the interconnectedness of all life.

Alternate Nostril Breathing (Nadi Sodhan): A pranayama (breathwork) practice that balances the flow of energy between the left and right hemispheres of the brain, harmonizing mind, body, and spirit through the breath.

Anxious Attachment Style: Characterized by a deep fear of abandonment and insecurity in relationships, individuals with this attachment style often seek constant reassurance and validation, experiencing heightened anxiety and sensitivity to perceived rejection or separation.

Asanas: Postures practiced in yoga that align with the body, mind, and spirit, promoting flexibility, strength, and inner balance.

Attachment Styles: Patterns of bonding and connection formed in early life, influencing our emotional and relational dynamics throughout our journey. These styles were extensively studied by John Bowlby in his series *Attachment and Loss* (1969–1980).

Attachment Theory: A framework explaining how our early connections with caregivers shape our relational experiences and emotional bonds throughout our lives, as explored by Mary Ainsworth in her "Strange Situation" study (1970).

Aura: The luminous electromagnetic field that surrounds your being, reflecting your energy, health, and spiritual essence.

Automatic Writing: A practice where the hand channels words from the subconscious mind, allowing the Soul's wisdom to flow onto the page. Helen Schucman's *A Course in Miracles* (published in 1976) is a well-known example of this practice.

Avoidant Attachment Style: Characterized by a strong desire for independence and self-reliance, individuals with this attachment style often avoid emotional intimacy and closeness, appearing distant or detached in relationships to protect themselves from potential rejection or vulnerability.

Ayahuasca: A revered plant medicine from the Amazon, used in sacred ceremonies to connect with higher realms, heal the spirit, and gain profound insights.

Belly Breathing: A grounding breath technique that engages the diaphragm, nurturing relaxation and infusing the body with vital life force energy. Breathing into the belly engages the parasympathetic nervous system and brings on a feeling of calmness, rest, and relaxation. This breathing technique is especially helpful for those feeling anxious.

Bessel van der Kolk: A psychiatrist and trauma specialist whose ground-breaking book *The Body Keeps the Score* (2014) explores how trauma impacts the body and mind, offering insights into healing through body-centered therapies.

Bottom of Your Exhale: The moment at the end of an exhalation where the lungs are empty, a space of deep surrender and connection to the earth.

Boundaries: Limits individuals set to protect themselves from manipulation, violation, or overuse. These boundaries determine acceptable behavior in physical, emotional, and mental interactions, helping maintain self-respect and well-being. They can be physical (personal space), emotional (sharing feelings), or mental (beliefs and thoughts). Clear boundaries ensure effective communication of needs and limits, fostering mutual respect and healthy relationships.

Breathwork: Techniques such as Holotropic breathwork (developed by Stanislav Grof in 1976), and rebirthing involve controlled breathing patterns to induce altered states of consciousness. Breathwork can promote relaxation, release emotional blockages, and guide you into opening the door to spiritual experiences.

Bufo (5-MeO-DMT): A potent entheogen derived from the secretion of the *Bufo alvarius* toad. Originating in the Sonoran Desert, it is used in shamanic practices to induce profound mystical experiences, ego dissolution, and deep spiritual insights. Its effects are rapid and intense, often leading to transformative healing.

Carl Jung: A visionary Swiss psychiatrist and founder of analytical psychology, known for his exploration of the collective unconscious and archetypes that shape our inner worlds. His book *Man and His Symbols* (1964) is a seminal work in this field.

Chakras: Spiritual energy centers within the body, originating from ancient Indian traditions. Each chakra corresponds to specific physical, emotional, and spiritual aspects of being. There are seven main chakras, aligned along the spine from the base to the crown, influencing overall health, energy flow, and consciousness.

Chant in three languages of consciousness: A sacred practice involving vocal tones to connect with different levels of existence:

- Human: Normal or loud voice (the world)
- Lovers: Strong whisper (longing to belong)
- Divine: Mentally; silent (Infinity)

Chest Breathing: Shallow breathing that confines the breath to the chest, often linked to stress and anxiety, and a call to reconnect with deeper, more nourishing breaths.

Clearing Space: The sacred practice of creating an orderly, harmonious environment by removing physical clutter and negative energies. This process prepares the mind and spirit for deep introspection, meditation, and spiritual work, fostering a sense of peace, safety, clarity, and focus.

Collective Unconscious: The shared reservoir of human experience and wisdom, a realm where universal archetypes and collective memories reside. Carl Jung's *The Archetypes and The Collective Unconscious* (1959) delves into this concept.

Default Mode Network (DMN): Neural networks in the brain that are active during rest and self-referential thoughts. Psychedelics, art making, and meditation disrupt the DMN, fostering reduced ego boundaries, enhanced creativity, and deep introspection. This disruption facilitates transformative experiences, self-discovery, and emotional healing by accessing non-ordinary states of consciousness. Neuroscientist Marcus Raichle extensively studied this network.

Deja-Vu: The ethereal sensation that a current experience has been lived before, a whisper from the Soul reminding us of the interconnectedness of time.

Diets and Restrictions: Dietary practices often undertaken to purify the body and mind, enhancing the effectiveness of spiritual and healing ceremonies.

Dissociating: A psychological defense mechanism where an individual disconnects from thoughts, feelings, or memories, often in response to trauma. This can result in a sense of detachment from reality, identity, or the body, and serves as a coping strategy to avoid emotional overwhelm and distress.

Dimethyltryptamine (DMT): A powerful naturally occurring psychedelic found in plants like Chacruna leaves (*Psychotria viridis*) used in the Ayahuasca brew, and animals like the Bufo toad. Known for inducing intense, short-lived visionary experiences and profound spiritual insights, it is often referred to as the "spirit molecule."

Donald Hebb: A pioneering Canadian psychologist known for his work in neuropsychology. His seminal book, *The Organization of Behavior* (1949), introduced "cells that fire together, wire together," foundational for understanding neural networks and synaptic plasticity. Hebb's work significantly shaped psychology, neuroscience, and cognitive science, influencing our understanding of brain function and behavior.

Dream Yoga: A mystical practice of engaging with dreams to explore the unconscious mind, as described by Swami Sivananda Radha in her book *Realities of the Dreaming Mind: The Practice of Dream Yoga* (1980). This practice transforms the dream state into a powerful tool for spiritual awakening and self-realization.

Drishti: In yoga and meditation, a focused gaze or point of concentration is used to direct and deepen attention during practice, helping to develop inner awareness and concentration.

Dysregulating: The inability to manage and control emotional responses, leading to intense and often overwhelming emotions. This state disrupts one's ability to function effectively, causing difficulties in maintaining mental and emotional balance. It often results from trauma, stress, or mental health conditions.

Ego Dissolution: A transcendental experience where the boundaries of the Self dissolve, merging with the infinite and experiencing unity with all.

EMDR: *Eye Movement Desensitization and Reprocessing*, a therapeutic approach developed by Francine Shapiro for processing trauma by using bilateral stimulation to facilitate the brain's natural healing process.

Emotional Blocks: Energetic barriers that hinder the free flow of emotions, often rooted in past traumas, and ready to be gently released.

Enmeshment: The blending of emotional boundaries in relationships, leading to a loss of individual identity and calling for separation and clarity.

Entheogen: A plant or substance used in sacred rituals to induce altered states of consciousness and connect with the spiritual realm.

Eugene Gendlin: A philosopher and psychologist who developed the Focusing technique, a body-centered approach to therapy that helps individuals connect with their inner knowing. His seminal work *Focusing* (1978) details this practice.

Eye Gaze: A technique to direct attention and deepen meditation, focusing the sight and spirit on a single point. Also referred to as a drishti.

Feminine Energy: The nurturing, intuitive, and receptive force that flows within all humans, embodying the divine feminine qualities.

Finger of Jupiter (Index Finger): In spiritual and yogic traditions, the index finger, also known as the "Finger of Jupiter," symbolizes wisdom, knowledge, and ambition. It is associated with the planet Jupiter, which governs expansion, growth, and prosperity. In various mudras (hand gestures) used in meditation and yoga, such as Gyan Mudra, touching the tip of the index finger to the thumb is believed to enhance concentration, invoke wisdom, and stimulate the energy associated with the higher mind and spiritual enlightenment.

Flow State: A mental state where an individual is fully immersed and engaged in an activity, experiencing a sense of effortless concentration and enjoyment. Time seems to fade away, and there is a deep focus and involvement in the task at hand. This state often leads to enhanced performance and creativity.

Focusing: A body-centered therapeutic approach developed by Eugene Gendlin that helps individuals connect with their inner knowing and process unresolved emotions. His seminal work *Focusing* (1978) outlines this method.

Gestalt Approach: A holistic therapeutic method that honors the present moment and the wholeness of an individual's experience. Fritz Perls' *Gestalt Therapy: Excitement and Growth in the Human Personality* (1951) is a foundational text in this field.

Good Parent Message: Affirmations and loving messages internalized from caregivers, nurturing a positive self-concept and emotional well-being.

Grounding Techniques: Practices that anchor the spirit in the present moment, establishing stability and a deep connection to the earth.

Gyan Mudra: A symbolic hand gesture in yoga and meditation where the pointer finger touches the thumb, channeling the energy of wisdom and knowledge. Touching the tip of the index finger to the thumb is believed to enhance concentration, invoke wisdom, and stimulate the energy associated with the higher mind and spiritual enlightenment.

Harm Reduction Approach: A strategy aimed at minimizing the negative consequences associated with certain behaviors, particularly substance use. It focuses on practical, compassionate methods to reduce harm rather than solely promoting abstinence, emphasizing safety, education, and support for individuals.

Hatha And Raj Yoga: Branches of yoga that cultivate physical alignment (Hatha) and the royal path of self-discipline and meditation (Raj), guiding the Soul to higher consciousness.

Higher Self: The divine aspect of one's being, connected to higher wisdom, spiritual guidance, and infinite potential.

Ibogaine: A sacred plant medicine from the African Iboga shrub, used in traditional ceremonies and modern healing for profound spiritual and therapeutic insights.

Icaros: Sacred songs sung by Amazonian Shamans or Cuenderos during Ayahuasca ceremonies believed to invoke spirits, ancestors, and healing energies, guiding, and protecting participants through their psychedelic journeys. Icaros play a crucial role in facilitating deep healing, spiritual connection, and transformation, integral to the ceremonial experience.

Ida: In yogic tradition, Ida is one of the three main nadis (energy channels) in the body, representing the lunar energy. It flows on the left side of the spine, associated with calmness, intuition, and the feminine aspect of consciousness.

IFS Model: Internal Family Systems, a therapeutic approach that recognizes the multiplicity of the mind, with each part holding unique perspectives and qualities. Richard C. Schwartz's *Internal Family Systems Therapy* (1995) elaborates on this model.

Indigenous: Referring to the original peoples of a region, their sacred traditions, and ancestral wisdom that connect us to the earth and spirit.

Inner Child: The pure, innocent aspect of oneself that retains the qualities, emotions, and memories of childhood, longing for love and healing.

Inner Power: The innate spiritual strength and resilience within each Soul, accessed through deep inner work and personal growth.

Integration Stages: The phases of processing and assimilating insights from psychedelic experiences. This process fosters lasting personal growth, emotional healing, and a deeper understanding of oneself.

Integrative Body Psychotherapy (IBP): A holistic therapeutic approach that weaves together physical, emotional, and mental processes to heal and harmonize the being. Jack Rosenberg's *Body, Self, and Soul: Sustaining Integration* (1985) provides insight into this method.

Intention: An aim set before embarking on a psychedelic journey, guiding the Soul's direction and focus toward higher consciousness and spiritual growth.

Jaguar Medicine (Synthetic 5-MeO-DMT): A powerful synthetic entheogen that mirrors the effects of natural 5-MeO-DMT found in the Buffo toad, guiding profound mystical journeys.

Jalandhar Bandh: A yoga practice involving a throat lock to control energy flow and deepen meditation. This is achieved by slightly lowering the chin to open up the back of the neck for Kundalini energy to move into the crown chakra.

Joan Kellogg: An esteemed Art Therapist who worked with Stan Grof. She is known for her work with mandalas, which she explored extensively in her book *Mandalas: Path of Beauty* (1977). Kellogg's work has illuminated the therapeutic power of creating and interpreting mandalas for self-discovery and healing. Using mandalas for reflection is still used within Holotropic Breathwork.

John Kabat-Zinn: A pioneer in mindfulness-based stress reduction (MBSR), integrating mindfulness meditation into mainstream medicine. His seminal work, *Wherever You Go, There You Are* (1994), teaches mindfulness techniques to reduce stress, enhance well-being, and promote emotional balance, revolutionizing how mindfulness is perceived and practiced in modern Western healthcare.

Joseph Tafur: A renowned doctor and shaman who bridges Western medicine and traditional shamanic healing, as detailed in his book *The Fellowship of the River* (2017).

Judith Herman: A psychiatrist renowned for her ground-breaking work on trauma and recovery. Her seminal book, *Trauma and Recovery*

(1992), established a comprehensive framework for understanding and treating trauma, emphasizing the importance of safety, remembrance, and reconnection. Herman's work revolutionized trauma healing by highlighting the profound impact of trauma on individuals and advocating for Trauma-informed care practices.

Kambo: A traditional Amazonian medicine derived from the secretions of the *Phyllomedusa bicolor frog*. Used in psychedelic therapy for its purgative and detoxifying properties, Kambo facilitates emotional and physical cleansing, often leading to profound healing and clarity by purging toxins and releasing emotional blockages.

Ketamine: A dissociative anesthetic now used in psychedelic therapy for its rapid antidepressant effects. Legal in many areas, it is administered in clinical settings to treat depression, PTSD, and anxiety. Clinics are opening up globally, offering supervised ketamine-assisted therapy to facilitate emotional and psychological healing.

Kundalini Energy: The coiled serpent of spiritual energy resting at the base of the spine, waiting to be awakened through sacred practices.

Kundalini Yoga: An ancient practice originating in India that combines aspects of both Hatha and Raj Yoga, focused on awakening the Kundalini energy coiled at the base of the spine. Combining postures (asanas), breathwork (pranayama), mudras (hand gestures), drishti (eye gazes), meditation, and chanting (mantras), it aims to promote spiritual enlightenment, heightened consciousness, and holistic well-being by channeling this powerful energy through the body's energy centers (chakras).

Limbic Region of The Brain: The emotional epicenter of the brain, where memories and feelings intertwine to shape our experiences.

Lysergic Acid Diethylamide (LSD): A powerful psychedelic that opens the mind to expansive realms of perception, thought, and emotion, first synthesized by Swiss Chemist Albert Hofmann in 1938 and discussed in his book *LSD: My Problem Child* (1980).

Macro dose: A high dosage of a psychedelic substance that induces a profound and intense altered state of consciousness. This level of dosing is used for deep therapeutic work and can lead to significant psychological insights, mystical experiences, and emotional breakthroughs.

Mandalas: Sacred geometric patterns (Sanskrit: "circle") representing the universe or Self, originating from Hindu and Buddhist traditions. Carl Jung and Joan Kellogg used mandalas for psychological analysis and healing. These patterns symbolize unity, balance, and cosmic order. Creating or contemplating mandalas promotes mindfulness, emotional stability, and a deeper connection to the Self and the cosmos.

Mantras: Sacred sounds and phrases repeated during meditation to focus the mind and invoke spiritual energy. They work to stimulate specific nadis (energy channels) in the body, enhancing neurochemical secretions like serotonin and dopamine, promoting relaxation, focus, and spiritual growth. Regular chanting balances the chakras, harmonizes the mind and body, and induces profound psychological and physiological benefits.

MAOI Medications: MAOIs enhance and prolong the effects of Psychedelics like DMT by preventing its breakdown. Interactions require caution due to risks of serotonin syndrome with SSRIs, hypertension with stimulants, and dangerous reactions with certain pain medications. Safe use involves consulting healthcare professionals, following dietary restrictions, proper dosages, safe environments, and having a support system.

Marcus Raichle: A neuroscientist who identified the Default Mode Network (DMN) in the brain, contributing significantly to our understanding of the brain's resting state and its role in self-referential thoughts and consciousness. His research has been foundational in the study of brain function and connectivity.

Martina Hoffmann: A visionary artist associated with **Stanislav Grof** and endorsed by **Albert Hofmann**, Martina Hoffmann explores themes of consciousness, transformation, and the feminine divine through her surreal and spiritually inspired artwork. She contributed to Grof's *Modern Consciousness Research and the Understanding of Art* and has participated in events honoring his work. Influenced by her late partner **Robert Venosa**, her art reflects the interplay between altered states and creative expression, making her a significant figure in the visionary art movement.

Masculine Energy: The assertive, logical, and action-oriented force within all humans, embodying the divine masculine qualities.

Meditation: Practices that quiet the mind and foster inner exploration, guiding the Soul into non-ordinary states of consciousness.

Mescaline: A sacred psychedelic found in certain cacti, known for its ability to induce visionary and spiritual experiences, as described in Aldous Huxley's *The Doors of Perception* (1954).

Michael Pollan: A journalist and author known for his exploration of Psychedelics and their potential to transform consciousness and heal the mind. His book *How to Change Your Mind* (2018) delves into the science and history of Psychedelics.

Micro-dose: Micro-dosing involves taking very small, sub-perceptual amounts of a psychedelic substance. This practice is intended to enhance cognitive function, creativity, and emotional balance without producing noticeable psychedelic effects. Typically, a micro-dose is about 1/10th to 1/20th of a standard dose.

Moon Energy: The gentle, reflective energy associated with the moon, symbolizing intuition, nurturing, and the divine feminine.

Mudra: A symbolic or ritual gesture commonly used in Hindu and Buddhist practices, particularly during meditation and yoga. These gestures are performed with the hands and fingers and are believed to influence the flow of energy within the body, enhancing physical, emotional, and spiritual well-being. Each mudra is associated with specific benefits and intentions.

Near Death Experience (NDE): A profound psychological event that typically occurs to individuals who are close to death or have been in situations of intense physical or emotional danger. Common features of NDEs include feelings of peace, out-of-body experiences, seeing a tunnel or light, and encounters with spiritual beings or deceased loved ones. These experiences often have a lasting impact on the individual's perception of life, death, and spirituality.

Neural Pathways: Connections between neurons in the brain that are strengthened through repeated use, forming the basis for habits, and learned behaviors. This concept was extensively studied by psychologist Donald Hebb, known for Hebbian theory.

Neurochemical: Pertaining to the chemicals in the brain that influence mood, behavior, and cognition.

Neurophysiological: Relating to the functions and activities of the nervous system and the brain.

Neuroplasticity: The brain's ability to reorganize itself by forming new neural connections. Altered states of consciousness can reroute neuropathways, supporting changes in behavior and habits.

Parasympathetic Engagement: Activation of the parasympathetic nervous system, which promotes relaxation and recovery.

Pat Ogden: One of the first key figures in somatic psychology and the founder of the Sensorimotor Psychotherapy Institute. Her book *Trauma and the Body* (2006) explores the integration of body and mind in trauma therapy.

Peter Levine: A trauma specialist and the creator of Somatic Experiencing, a body-focused approach to healing trauma. His book *Waking the Tiger: Healing Trauma* (1997) is a seminal work in this field.

Pineal Gland: Often referred to as the "third eye," this gland regulates sleep-wake cycles by producing melatonin. Spiritually, it is considered a gateway to higher consciousness and spiritual insight, facilitating deep meditation and mystical experiences. Ancient practices emphasize its activation for spiritual enlightenment and connection to the divine.

Pingala: In yogic tradition, Pingala is one of the three main nadis (energy channels) in the body, representing solar energy. It flows on the right side of the spine, associated with activity, logic, and the masculine aspect of consciousness. Pingala balances Ida's lunar energy, promoting a harmonious flow of life force.

Pituitary Gland: Known as the "master gland," it regulates vital hormones influencing growth, metabolism, and reproduction. In meditation, it is believed to enhance intuition and spiritual awareness, often associated with the third eye chakra. It plays a crucial role in achieving spiritual enlightenment and higher states of consciousness.

Plasticine: A non-drying, malleable clay used for modeling and sculpting. Originating in the late 19th century, it is made from calcium salts, petroleum jelly, and aliphatic acids. Plasticine is popular in Art

Therapy, animation, and children's play for its versatility, allowing users to create and reshape figures repeatedly without hardening.

Play-Doh: A popular modeling compound brand by Hasbro, made from a non-toxic mixture of water, salt, and flour. Known for its vibrant colors, it is used for children's creative and educational activities.

Prana: Prana is the Sanskrit term for "life force" or "vital energy" that permeates the universe. It is considered the essence of life and consciousness, flowing through the body's energy channels (nadis) and centers (chakras). In yoga and meditation, controlling prana enhances physical, mental, and spiritual well-being.

Pranayama: An ancient yogic practice involving breath control techniques to enhance physical, mental, and spiritual well-being. Derived from Sanskrit words "prana" (life force) and "ayama" (control), pranayama regulates energy flow, calms the mind, and prepares for meditation.

Primary Scenario Arena: In Integrative Body Psychotherapy, this is the conceptual space where foundational life experiences and core beliefs are formed. Early interactions with caregivers and significant events shape one's worldview, emotional responses, and behaviors, aiding in deep personal growth and healing.

Protectors: The Managers: Parts of the psyche that work to prevent emotional pain by managing behaviors and environments proactively.

Protectors in IFS: In Internal Family Systems (IFS), developed by Dick Schwartz, protectors are parts of the psyche that defend against emotional pain. IFS sees these protectors as essential to understanding and healing the internal system

- Proactive: Managers: These protectors aim to prevent harm by controlling daily life, maintaining order, and avoiding situations that might trigger emotional distress. They keep the person functional and organized.
- Reactive: Firefighters: These protectors act impulsively to extinguish emotional pain when it arises. They engage in behaviors like substance use, overeating, or distraction to quickly numb or escape from overwhelming feelings.

Psychedelic Art: Art that is inspired by, influenced by, or derives from Psychedelics or non-ordinary states of consciousness. It captures the visual intensity, mystery, beauty, and sense of transcendence that can be experienced in altered states of consciousness.

Psycho-Education: The process of educating individuals about psychological concepts and practices to enhance their understanding and coping skills.

Psycholytic Dose: Refers to a moderate dosage of a psychedelic substance that induces a mild to moderate altered state of consciousness. This level of dosage allows for therapeutic exploration and insight without overwhelming the individual, facilitating introspection and emotional release.

Psychotropic: Relating to substances that affect the mind, mood, or behavior.

Richard Schwartz: The developer of the Internal Family Systems (IFS) model, which recognizes the multiplicity of the mind with each part holding unique perspectives and qualities. His book *Internal Family Systems Therapy* (1995) elaborates on this model.

Sacred Geometry: Describes the architecture of the universe and the patterns that are the building blocks of everything in life, from plants and stars to atoms and cells. It involves geometric shapes that symbolize the interconnectedness and unity of all things.

Sanskrit: An ancient Indic language of India, in which the Hindu scriptures and classical Indian epic poems are written and from which many northern Indian languages are derived.

Secure Attachment Style: A healthy attachment pattern characterized by trust, emotional closeness, and a positive view of oneself and others.

Self-Regulate: The ability to manage and control one's emotions, behaviors, and physiological responses, especially in stressful situations.

Serotonergic Medications: Drugs that affect serotonin levels in the brain, often used to treat depression and anxiety.

Serotonin: A neurotransmitter that plays a key role in mood regulation, sleep, and overall well-being.

Serotonin Syndrome: A potentially life-threatening condition caused by excessive levels of serotonin in the brain, often due to drug interactions.

Set And Setting: Psychological and environmental factors that influence the psychedelic experience. "Set" encompasses the mindset, intentions, beliefs, and emotional state of the individual. "Setting" includes the physical environment, social context, and interpersonal dynamics.

Shuni Mudra: A hand gesture where the middle finger touches the thumb, symbolizing patience and discipline.

Somatic: Relating to the body, especially as distinct from the mind, often used in the context of body-centered therapies.

Soul: The spiritual essence of a person, often considered eternal and the core of one's being.

Soul's Path: The unique journey and purpose of an individual's Soul, encompassing their experiences, growth, and destiny.

SSRI Antidepressants: Selective Serotonin Reuptake Inhibitors, a class of medications commonly prescribed to treat depression and anxiety.

Stanislav Grof: A psychiatrist and pioneer in the field of transpersonal psychology and psychedelic therapy. His work with LSD therapy and development of Holotropic Breathwork are chronicled in his books *LSD Psychotherapy* (1980) and *The Holotropic Mind* (1992).

Stimulants: Substances that increase activity in the nervous system, leading to increased alertness, energy, and mood elevation.

Subtle Bodies: Layers of energy fields that surround and interpenetrate the physical body, according to various spiritual traditions.

Sun Energy: The vibrant, active, and energizing force associated with the sun, often linked to masculine qualities.

Swami Sivananda Radha: A yogini and author who brought the practice of Dream Yoga to the West. Her book *Realities of the Dreaming Mind: The Practice of Dream Yoga* (1980) provides a comprehensive guide to using dreams for spiritual awakening and self-realization.

Sympathetic System Engagement: Activation of the sympathetic nervous system, which prepares the body for action and stress responses.

Synthetic Psychedelic: Psychedelic drugs synthesized in laboratories to mimic the effects of naturally occurring substances, such as LSD, MDMA, and 2C-B.

Top of the Inhale: The point at the peak of an inhalation where the lungs are fully expanded, often used in breathing exercises to enhance focus and mindfulness.

Transcendental Meditation (TM): A form of silent mantra meditation designed to promote relaxation, self-development, and stress relief through the repetition of a specific sound or mantra, as taught by Maharishi Mahesh Yogi in The Science of Being and Art of Living (1963).

Transpersonal: Pertaining to experiences or aspects of the psyche that transcend the individual and connect to a greater collective or spiritual dimension.

Trauma-Informed Therapy: An approach that recognizes the impact of trauma on mental, emotional, and physical well-being, promoting safety, empowerment, and choice to avoid re-traumatization.

Visualization: A technique involving the use of mental imagery to achieve relaxation, healing, or enhanced performance.

Yoga Nidra: A guided meditation practice often referred to as "yogic sleep" that aims to achieve deep relaxation and awareness through a series of guided visualizations and body scans. Swami Satyananda Saraswati's *Yoga Nidra* (1976) details this practice.

Yogic Science: The study and practice of yoga, encompassing its physical, mental, and spiritual aspects to promote overall well-being and enlightenment.

Zen: A school of Mahayana Buddhism that emphasizes meditation and intuition rather than ritual and scripture, aiming for a direct experience of enlightenment, as explored by D.T. Suzuki in *Zen Mind, Beginner's Mind* (1970).

REFERENCES

Adams, K. (2016). *Journal to the Self: Twenty-Two Paths to Personal Growth.* Grand Central Publishing.

Ainsworth, M. D., & Bowlby, J. (1991). An Ethological Approach to Personality Development. *American Psychologist, 46*(4), 333–341. https://doi.org/10.1037/0003-066X.46.4.333

Allione, T. (2008). *Feeding Your Demons: Ancient Wisdom for Resolving Inner Conflict.* Little, Brown and Company.

Alper, K. R. (2001). Ibogaine: A Review. *The Alkaloids: Chemistry and Biology, 56*, 1–38.

Anzaldúa, G. (1987). *Borderlands/La Frontera: The New Mestiza.* Aunt Lute Books.

Assay, D., Lee Rosenberg, J., & Rand, M. (1987a). *Body, Self, and Soul: Sustaining Integration.* Humanics Publishing Group.

Assay, L., Rosenberg, J. L., & Rand, R. (1987b). *Integrative Body Psychotherapy: Toward a Comprehensive Understanding of the Whole Person.* North Atlantic Books.

Beaty, R. E., et al. (2015). Default and Executive Network Coupling Supports Creative Idea Production. *Scientific Reports, 5*, 10964. https://doi.org/10.1038/srep10964

Bessel van der Kolk. (2014). *The Body Keeps the Score: Brain, Mind, and Body in the Healing of Trauma.* Viking Press.

Beyer, S. V. (2009). *Singing to the Plants: A Guide to Mestizo Shamanism in the Upper Amazon.* University of New Mexico Press.

Bolwerk, A., et al. (2014). How Art Changes Your Brain: Differential Effects of Visual Art Production and Cognitive Art Evaluation on Functional Brain Connectivity. *PLOS ONE, 9*(7), e101035. https://doi.org/10.1371/journal.pone.0101035

Bowlby, J. (1988). *A Secure Base: Parent-Child Attachment and Healthy Human Development.* Basic Books.

Boyer, E. W., & Shannon, M. (2005). The Serotonin Syndrome. *New England Journal of Medicine, 352*(11), 1112–1120.

Bradford, C. (2020). *The Age of Aquarius: A Global Shift.* New Earth Publishing.

Brantley, J., McKay, M., & Wood, J. C. (2007). *The Dialectical Behavior Therapy Skills Workbook: Practical DBT Exercises for Learning Mindfulness, Interpersonal Effectiveness, Emotion Regulation, and Distress Tolerance.* New Harbinger Publications.

Braud, W. (2003). *Distant Mental Influence: Its Contributions to Science, Healing, and Human Interactions*. Hampton Roads Publishing.

Brewer, J. A., et al. (2011). Meditation Experience Is Associated with Differences in Default Mode Network Activity and Connectivity. *Proceedings of the National Academy of Sciences, 108*(50), 20254–20259.

Briere, J. (2002). *Treating Adult Survivors of Severe Childhood Abuse and Neglect: Further Development of an Integrative Model*. Sage Publications.

Brown, B. (2017). *Braving the Wilderness: The Quest for True Belonging and the Courage to Stand Alone*. Random House.

Brown, B. (2010). *The Gifts of Imperfection: Let Go of Who You Think You're Supposed to Be and Embrace Who You Are*. Hazelden Publishing.

Brown, R., & Gerbarg, P. (2012). *The Healing Power of the Breath: Simple Techniques to Reduce Stress and Anxiety, Enhance Concentration, and Balance Your Emotions*. Shambhala Publications.

Callahan, M. J. (2016). *Mindfulness Based Art: The SPARKS Guide for Educators and Counselors*. Friesen Press.

Cameron, J. (1992). *The Artist's Way: A Spiritual Path to Higher Creativity*. Penguin Books.

Campbell, J. (2016). *The Hero's Journey: Joseph Campbell on His Life and Work*. New World Library.

Capacchione, L. (1988). *The Power of Your Other Hand: A Course in Channeling the Inner Wisdom of the Right Brain*. Tarcher/Putnam.

Carhart-Harris, R. L., Bolstridge, M., Rucker, J., Day, C. M., Erritzoe, D., Kaelen, M., Bloomfield, M. A., Rickard, J. A., Forbes, B., Feilding, A., Taylor, D., Pilling, S., Curran, V., & Nutt, D. J. (2016). Psilocybin with Psychological Support for Treatment-Resistant Depression: An Open-Label Feasibility Study. *The Lancet Psychiatry, 3*(7), 619–627. https://doi.org/10.1016/s2215-0366(16)30065-7

Carhart-Harris, R. L., & Friston, K. J. (2019). REBUS and the Anarchic Brain: Toward a Unified Model of the Brain Action of Psychedelics. *Pharmacological Reviews, 71*(3), 316–344.

Carhart-Harris, R. L., & Goodwin, G. M. (2017). The Therapeutic Potential of Psychedelic Drugs: Past, Present, and Future. *Neuropsychopharmacology, 42*(11), 2105–2113.

Carhart-Harris, R. L., & Nutt, D. J. (2017). Psychedelics in the Treatment of Anxiety, Depression and Addiction. *Neuropharmacology, 142*, 98–108.

Carhart-Harris, R. L., et al. (2012). Neural Correlates of the Psychedelic State as Determined by fMRI Studies with Psilocybin. *Proceedings of the National Academy of Sciences, 109*(6), 2138–2143.

Carhart-Harris, R. L., et al. (2014). The Entropic Brain: A Theory of Conscious States Informed by Neuroimaging Research with Psychedelic Drugs. *Frontiers in Human Neuroscience, 8*, 20.

Carhart-Harris, R. L., et al. (2018a). Psychedelic Experience Alters Neural Processes Underlying Empathy. *Neuroscience & Biobehavioral Reviews, 92*, 294–308.

Carhart-Harris, R. L., et al. (2018b). Psychedelic Therapy: A Roadmap for Future Research and Practice. *Current Opinion in Psychiatry, 31*(1), 38–45.

Carhart-Harris, R. L., et al. (2018c). Increased Nature Relatedness and Decreased Authoritarian Political Views After Psilocybin Use. *Journal of Psychopharmacology, 32*(8), 811–819.

Carhart-Harris, R. L., Roseman, L., Bolstridge, M., Demetriou, L., Pannekoek, J. N., Wall, M. B., ... & Nutt, D. J. (2017). Psilocybin for Treatment-Resistant Depression: fMRI-measured Brain Mechanisms. *Scientific Reports, 8*(1), 1–10.

Carpendale, M. (2009). *Essence and Praxis in the Art Therapy Studio*. Trafford Publishing.

Carpendale, M. (2021). *A Geography of Dream Work and Art Therapy*. Kindle Direct Publishing.

Carpendale, M. (2023). *The Magpie's Nest: Arts-Based Supervision*. Essenze Publications.

Case, C., & Dalley, T. (2014). *The Handbook of Art Therapy*. Routledge.

Chu, P. S. K., Kwok, S. C., Lam, K. M., Chu, T. Y., Chan, S. W., Man, C. W., ... & Tsui, K. L. (2008). 'Street Ketamine'–Associated Bladder Dysfunction: A Report of Ten Cases. *Hong Kong Medical Journal, 14*(1), 84–85.

Clear, J. (2018). *Atomic Habits: An Easy & Proven Way to Build Good Habits & Break Bad Ones*. Avery.

Cott, A. (1995). *Fasting: The Ultimate Diet*. Healing Arts Press.

Courtois, C. A. (2004). Complex Trauma, Complex Reactions: Assessment and Treatment. *Psychotherapy: Theory, Research, Practice, Training, 41*(4), 412–425.

Courtois, C. A., & Ford, J. D. (2013). *Treating Complex Traumatic Stress Disorders: Scientific Foundations and Therapeutic Models*. Guilford Press.

Csikszentmihalyi, M. (1990). *Flow: The Psychology of Optimal Experience*. Harper & Row.

Davidson, R. J., Kabat-Zinn, J., Schumacher, J., Rosenkranz, M., Muller, D., Santorelli, S. F., ... & Sheridan, J. F. (2003). Alterations in Brain and Immune Function Produced by Mindfulness Meditation. *Psychosomatic Medicine, 65*(4), 564–570.

Davidson, R. J., & Lutz, A. (2008). Buddha's Brain: Neuroplasticity and Meditation. *IEEE Signal Processing Magazine, 25*(1), 176–174.

Davidson, R. J., & McEwen, B. S. (2012). Social Influences on Neuroplasticity: Stress and Interventions to Promote Well-Being. *Nature Neuroscience, 15*(5), 689–695. https://doi.org/10.1038/nn.3093

Davis, A. K., Barsuglia, J. P., Lancelotta, R., Grant, R. M., & Renn, E. (2019). The Epidemiology of 5-methoxy-N,N-dimethyltryptamine (5-MeO-DMT) Use: Benefits, Consequences, Patterns of Use, and Abuse Potential. *Journal of Psychopharmacology, 33*(9), 1018–1030.

den Brave, P. S., Bruins, E., & Bronkhorst, M. W. (2014). Phyllomedusa bicolor Skin Secretion and the Kambô Ritual. *Journal of Venomous Animals and Toxins Including Tropical Diseases, 20*(1), 40.

Dobkin de Rios, M. (1984). *Hallucinogens, Cross-Cultural Perspectives*. University of New Mexico Press.

Dobkin de Rios, M., & Janiger, O. (2003). *LSD, Spirituality, and the Creative Process: Based on the Groundbreaking Research of Oscar Janiger, M.D.* Inner Traditions / Bear & Co.

Dobkin de Rios, M., & Rumrrill, R. (2008). *A Hallucinogenic Tea, Laced with Controversy: Ayahuasca in the Amazon and the United States*. Praeger.

Doblin, R., et al. (2019). MDMA-Assisted Psychotherapy for PTSD: A Phase 3 Trial. *Nature Medicine, 25*(1), 1–8.

Domhoff, G. W. (2003). *The Scientific Study of Dreams: Neural Networks, Cognitive Development, and Content Analysis*. American Psychological Association.

Dore, J., Turnipseed, B., Dwyer, S., Turnipseed, A., Andries, J., Ascani, G., Monnette, C., Huidekoper, A., Strauss, N., Wolfson, P., & Hamilton, S. (2019). Ketamine Assisted Psychotherapy (KAP): Patient Demographics, Clinical Data, and Outcomes in Three Large Practices Administering Ketamine with Psychotherapy. *Journal of Psychoactive Drugs, 51*(2), 189–198. https://doi.org/10.1080/02791072.2019.1587556

Dossey, L. (2001). *Healing Beyond the Body: Medicine and the Infinite Reach of the Mind*. Shambhala Publications.

Dyson, P. S. (2020). *Premka: White Bird in a Golden Cage: My Life with Yogi Bhajan*. Eyes Wide Publishing.

Eliade, M. (1958). *Rites and Symbols of Initiation*. Harper & Row.

Eliade, M. (1964). *Shamanism: Archaic Techniques of Ecstasy*. Princeton University Press.

Erikson, E. H. (1950). *Childhood and Society*. W. W. Norton & Company.

Fadiman, J. (2011). *The Psychedelic Explorer's Guide: Safe, Therapeutic, and Sacred Journeys*. Park Street Press.

Falconer, R. (2023). *The Others Within Us: Internal Family Systems, Porous Mind, and Spirit Possession*. Great Mystery Press.

Feuerstein, G. (1998). *The Yoga Tradition: Its History, Literature, Philosophy, and Practice*. Hohm Press.

Feuerstein, G. (2001). *The Yoga Tradition: Its History, Literature, Philosophy and Practice*. Hohm Press.

Fikes, J. C. (1996). *Rebirth and Regeneration in the Peyote Way: Symbolic Healing in Huichol Ritual*. The University of Arizona Press.

Fincher, S. (2010). *Creating Mandalas: For Insight, Healing, and Self-Expression*. Shambhala Publications.

Fireside Project. (n.d.). Psychedelic Peer Support Line. Retrieved from Fireside Project website. https://firesideproject.org.

Ford, D. (2017). *The Dark Side of the Light Chasers: Reclaiming Your Power, Creativity, Brilliance, and Dreams*. Penguin Books.

Forte, R. (Ed.). (1997). *Entheogens and the Future of Religion*. Council on Spiritual Practices.

Fotiou, E. (2016). The Globalization of Ayahuasca Shamanism and the Erasure of Indigenous Cultures. *Anthropological Quarterly, 89*(3), 803–831.

Fotiou, E. (2020). The Role of Indigenous Knowledges in Psychedelic Science. *Journal of Psychedelic Studies, 4*(1), 16–23.

Franklin, M. (2017). *Art as Contemplative Practice: Expressive Pathways to the Self*. State University of New York Press.

Freud, S. (1900). *The Interpretation of Dreams*. Macmillan.

Freud, S. (1923). *The Ego and the Id*. The Standard Edition of the Complete Psychological Works of Sigmund Freud, Volume XIX (1923–1925): The Ego and the Id and Other Works.

Ganim, B., & Fox, S. (1999). *Visual Journaling: Going Deeper than Words*. Quest Books.

Garcia-Romeu, A., Griffiths, R. R., & Johnson, M. W. (2014). Psilocybin-Occasioned Mystical Experiences in the Treatment of Tobacco Addiction. *Current Drug Abuse Reviews, 7*(3), 157–164.

Garrison, K. A., et al. (2015). Meditators and Non-Meditators Exhibit Differences in Default Mode Network Connectivity during Resting State. *Neuroscience Letters, 571*, 52–57.

Gasser, P., et al. (2014). Safety and Efficacy of Lysergic Acid Diethylamide-Assisted Psychotherapy for Anxiety Associated with Life-threatening Diseases. *Journal of Nervous and Mental Disease, 202*(7), 513–520.

Gazzaniga, M. S. (2000). Cerebral Specialization and Interhemispheric Communication. *Brain, 123*(7), 1293–1326.

Gendlin, E. T. (1978). *Focusing*. Bantam Books.

George, J. R., Michaels, T. I., Sevelius, J., & Williams, M. T. (2020). The Psychedelic Renaissance and the Limitations of a White-Dominant Medical Framework: A Call for Indigenous and Ethnic Minority Inclusion. *Journal of Psychedelic Studies, 4*(1), 4–15.

Gilbert, P. (2014). *The Compassionate Mind: A New Approach to Facing the Challenges of Life*. New Harbinger.

Goleman, D. (2006). *Social Intelligence: The New Science of Human Relationships*. Bantam Books.

Gomez, A. (2020). *Shamanism and Indigenous Struggles in the Amazon*. Indigenous Studies Press.

Gordon, A. (2018). *Ghostly Matters: Haunting and the Sociological Imagination*. University of Minnesota Press.

Gorman, E. M. (2018). *Harm Reduction in Substance Use and High-Risk Behaviour.* Routledge.

Gorman, I., Nielson, E. M., & Phelps, J. (2021). Psychedelic Harm Reduction and Integration: A Tool for Clinicians. *Journal of Psychedelic Studies, 4*(1), 5–18.

Goswami, S. (1999). *Layayoga: The Definitive Guide to the Chakras and Kundalini.* Inner Traditions.

Graveline, F. J. (1998). *Circle Works: Transforming Eurocentric Consciousness.* Fernwood Publishing.

Griffiths, R. R., et al. (2016). Psilocybin Produces Substantial and Sustained Decreases in Depression and Anxiety in Patients with Life-threatening Cancer: A Randomized Double-Blind Trial. *Journal of Psychopharmacology, 30*(12), 1181–1197.

Griffiths, R. R., Richards, W. A., McCann, U., & Jesse, R. (2008). Psilocybin can Occasion Mystical-type Experiences having Substantial and Sustained Personal Meaning and Spiritual Significance. *Psychopharmacology, 187*(3), 268–283.

Grof, S. (1976). *Realms of the Human Unconscious: Observations from LSD Research.* Viking Press.

Grof, S. (1980a). *LSD Psychotherapy: Exploring the Frontiers of the Hidden Mind.* Hunter House Publishers.

Grof, S. (1980b). *Realms of the Human Unconscious: Observations from LSD Research.* Viking Press.

Grof, S. (1985). *Beyond the Brain: Birth, Death, and Transcendence in Psychotherapy.* State University of New York Press.

Grof, S. (1993). *The Holotropic Mind: The Three Levels of Human Consciousness and How They Shape Our Lives.* HarperCollins.

Grof, S. (1997). *The Cosmic Game: Explorations of the Frontiers of Human Consciousness.* State University of New York Press.

Grof, S. (2000). *Psychology of the Future: Lessons from Modern Consciousness Research.* State University of New York Press.

Grof, S. (2008a). *LSD Psychotherapy: Exploring the Frontiers of the Hidden Mind.* Multidisciplinary Association for Psychedelic Studies.

Grof, S. (2008b). *The Ultimate Journey: Consciousness and the Mystery of Death.* Multidisciplinary Association for Psychedelic Studies (MAPS).

Grof, S. (2015). *Modern Consciousness Research and the Understanding of Art: Including the Visionary World of H.R. Giger.* Multidisciplinary Association for Psychedelic Studies.

Grof, S., & Halifax, J. (1977). *The Human Encounter with Death.* E.P. Dutton.

Guzmán, G. (2012). New Taxonomical and Ethnomycological Observations on *Psilocybe* s.s. (Fungi, Basidiomycota, Agaricomycetidae, Agaricales, Strophariaceae) from Mexico, Africa and Spain. *Acta Botánica Mexicana, 100*, 79–106. https://doi.org/10.21829/abm100.2012.32

Harman, W., & Rheingold, H. (1984*). Higher Creativity: Liberating the Unconscious for Breakthrough Insights.* Jeremy P. Tarcher.

Harner, M. J. (1990). *The Way of the Shaman.* Harper & Row.

Harris, M., & Fallot, R. D. (2001). *Using Trauma Theory to Design Service Systems.* Jossey-Bass.

Harris, R. (2015). *The Happiness Trap: How to Stop Struggling and Start Living.* Shambhala.

Harris, R. (2019a). *The Art of Mindful Living: Bringing Authenticity and Inner Wisdom into Your Daily Practice.* New Harbinger Publications.

Harris, R. (2019b). *The Happiness Trap: How to Stop Struggling and Start Living.* Shambhala Publications.

Hartmann, E. (1998). *Dreams and Nightmares: The New Theory on the Origin and Meaning of Dreams.* Plenum Press.

Hartogsohn, I. (2016). Set and Setting, Psychedelics, and the Placebo Response: An Extra-pharmacological Perspective on Psychopharmacology. *Journal of Psychopharmacology, 30*(12), 1259–1267.

Hazan, C., & Shaver, P. (1987). Romantic Love Conceptualized as an Attachment Process. *Journal of Personality and Social Psychology, 52*(3), 511–524.

Hebb, D. O. (1949). *The Organization of Behavior: A Neuropsychological Theory.* Wiley.

Herman, J. L. (1992). *Trauma and Recovery: The Aftermath of Violence—From Domestic Abuse to Political Terror.* Basic Books.

Hill, C. E. (2017). *Dream work in therapy: Facilitating exploration, Insight, and Action.* American Psychological Association.

Hillman, J. (1975). *Re-Visioning Psychology.* Harper & Row.

Hillman, J. (1979). *The Dream and the Underworld.* Harper & Row.

Hinz, L. D. (2009). *Expressive Therapies Continuum: A Framework for Using Art in Therapy.* Routledge.

Hofmann, A. (1980). *LSD: My Problem Child.* McGraw-Hill.

Holecek, A. (2016). *Dream Yoga: Illuminating Your Life through Lucid Dreaming and the Tibetan Yogas of Sleep.* Sounds True.

Holmes, J. (2014). *John Bowlby and Attachment Theory* (2nd ed.). Routledge.

Husum, C. (2023). *Sacred Geometry Visionary Art: Coloring Book.* Charmaine Husum.

Iacoboni, M. (2009). *Mirroring People: The New Science of How We Connect with Others.* Farrar, Straus and Giroux.

Immergut, M., & Yates Culadasa, J. (2017). *The Mind Illuminated: A Complete Meditation Guide Integrating Buddhist Wisdom and Brain Science for Greater Mindfulness.* Touchstone.

Johnson, M. W. (2018). Psychiatry Might Need Some Psychedelic Therapy. *Nature Medicine, 24*(4), 376–377. https://doi.org/10.1038/nm0418-376

Johnson, S. M. (2008). *Hold Me Tight: Seven Conversations for a Lifetime of Love.* Little, Brown & Co.

James, W. (1902/2002). *The Varieties of Religious Experience: A Study in Human Nature.* Routledge.

Johnson, M. W., Richards, W. A., & Griffiths, R. R. (2008). Human Hallucinogen Research: Guidelines for Safety. *Journal of Psychopharmacology, 22*(6), 603–620.

Johnson, R. A. (1986). *Inner Work: Using Dreams and Active Imagination for Personal Growth.* HarperOne.

Johnson, S. M. (2008). *Hold Me Tight: Seven Conversations for a Lifetime of Love.* Little, Brown Spark.

Jordan, M., & Hinds, J. (2016). *Ecotherapy: Theory, Research and Practice.* Macmillan International Higher Education.

Judith, A. (2001). *Eastern Body, Western Mind: Psychology and the Chakra System as a Path to the Self.* Celestial Arts.

Jung, C. G. (1933). *Modern Man in Search of a Soul.* Harcourt, Brace & World, Inc.

Jung, C. G. (1938). *Psychology and Religion: West and East.* Routledge & Kegan Paul.

Jung, C. G. (1953). *The Collected Works of C. G. Jung* (Vol. 9). Princeton University Press.

Jung, C. G. (1959). *The Archetypes and the Collective Unconscious.* Princeton University Press.

Jung, C. G. (1964). *Man and His Symbols.* Doubleday.

Jung, C. G. (1966). *The Practice of Psychotherapy: Essays on the Psychology of the Transference and Other Subjects* (Vol. 16). Princeton University Press.

Jung, C. G. (1969a). *Archetypes and the Collective Unconscious.* Princeton University Press.

Jung, C. G. (1969b). *The Collected Works of C. G. Jung: Volume 9 (Part 1).* Princeton University Press.

Jung, C. G. (1969c). *The Structure and Dynamics of the Psyche*. Princeton University Press.

Jung, C. G. (1973). *Mandala Symbolism*. Princeton University Press.

Jung, C. G. (1974). *Dreams*. Princeton University Press.

Jung, C. G. (1979). *Aion: Researches into the Phenomenology of the Self*. Princeton University Press

Jung, C. G. (2009). *The Red Book: Liber Novus* (S. Shamdasani, Ed.; M. Kyburz, J. Peck, & S. Shamdasani, Trans.). W. W. Norton & Company.

Kabat-Zinn, J. (1990). *Full Catastrophe Living: Using the Wisdom of Your Body and Mind to Face Stress, Pain, and Illness*. Delacorte Press.

Kabat-Zinn, J. (1994). *Wherever You Go, There You Are: Mindfulness Meditation in Everyday Life*. Hachette Books.

Kabat-Zinn, J. (2005). *Coming to Our Senses: Healing Ourselves and the World Through Mindfulness*. Hyperion.

Kaelen, M., et al. (2018). The Hidden Therapist: Evidence for a Central Role of Music in Psychedelic Therapy. *Psychopharmacology, 235*(2), 505–519.

Kellogg, J., Mac Rae, M., Bonny, H. L., & Di Leo, F. (1977). The Use of the Mandala in Psychological Evaluation and Treatment. *American Journal of Art Therapy, 16*(4), 123–134

Kellogg, J. (1992). *Mandala: Path of Beauty*. Williamsburg, VA: Graphic Publishing.

Khalsa, S. B., Cohen, L., McCall, T., Telles, S., Cramer, H. (2024). *The Principles and Practice of Yoga in Health Care*. Handspring Publishing.

Kirmayer, L. J. (2004). The cultural diversity of healing: Meaning, metaphor, and mechanism. *British Medical Bulletin, 69*(1), 33–48.

Kleinman, A. (1980). *Patients and Healers in the Context of Culture*. University of California Press.

Kornfield, J. (2009). *The Wise Heart: A Guide to the Universal Teachings of Buddhist Psychology*. Bantam Books.

Krippner, S. (1994). *Altered States of Consciousness*. Psychology Press.

Krystal, J. H., Karper, L. P., Seibyl, J. P., Freeman, G. K., Delaney, R., Bremner, J. D., … & Charney, D. S. (1994). Subanesthetic Effects of the Noncompetitive NMDA Antagonist, Ketamine, in Humans. Psychotomimetic, Perceptual, Cognitive, and Neuroendocrine Responses. *Archives of General Psychiatry, 51*(3), 199–214.

Labate, B. C., & Cavnar, C. (2014). *The Therapeutic Use of Ayahuasca*. Springer.

Labate, B. C., & Feeney, K. (2012). Ayahuasca and the Process of Regulation in Brazil and Beyond. *International Journal of Drug Policy, 23*(2), 154–161.

LaBerge, S., & Rheingold, H. (1990). *Exploring the World of Lucid Dreaming*. Ballantine Books.

LaChance, S. (2012). Automatic Writing and How to Tune into the Inner Self. *Journal of Spirituality Studies, 4*(2), 45–58.

Laderman, C., & Roseman, M. (1996). *The Performance of Healing*. Routledge.

Lajoux, J.-D. (1963). *The Rock Paintings of the Tassili*. World Publishing.

Lakoff, G., & Johnson, M. (1980). *Metaphors We Live By*. University of Chicago Press.

Layton, E. (1984). *Through the Looking Glass: Drawings by Elizabeth Layton*. Kansas City Southern Industries.

Leary, T., et al. (1963). The Psychedelic Experience: A Manual based on the Tibetan Book of the Dead. *Psychological Reports, 13*, 151–172.

Leary, T., Metzner, R., & Alpert, R. (1964). *The Psychedelic Experience: A Manual Based on the Tibetan Book of the Dead*. Citadel Press.

Lebedev, A. V., et al. (2015). Finding the Self by Losing the Self: Neural Correlates of Ego-Dissolution under Psilocybin. *Human Brain Mapping, 36*(8), 3137–3153. https://doi.org/10.1002/hbm.22833

Lévi-Strauss, C. (1963). *Structural Anthropology*. Basic Books.

Levine, P. A. (2010). *In an Unspoken Voice: How the Body Releases Trauma and Restores Goodness*. North Atlantic Books.

Levine, P. A. (2015). *Trauma and Memory: Brain and Body in a Search for the Living Past: A Practical Guide for Understanding and Working with Traumatic Memory*. North Atlantic Books.

Levine, P., & Frederick, A. (1997). *Waking the Tiger: Healing Trauma*. North Atlantic Books.

Levine, P., & Frederick, A. (2005). *Healing Trauma: A Pioneering Program for Restoring the Wisdom of Your Body*. Sounds True.

Levine, P., & Heller, D. (2010). *Attached: The New Science of Adult Attachment and How It Can Help You Find—and Keep—Love*. TarcherPerigee.

Liotti, G. (2004). Trauma, Dissociation, and Disorganized Attachment: Three Strands of a Single Braid. *Psychotherapy: Theory, Research, Practice, Training, 41*(4), 472–486.

Luna, L. E. (1984a). *Healing Practices in the Upper Amazon*. University of California Press.

Luna, L. E. (1984b). The Healing Practices of a Peruvian Shaman. *Journal of Ethnopharmacology, 11*(2), 123–133.

Luna, L. E., & Amaringo, P. (1999). *Ayahuasca Visions: The Religious Iconography of a Peruvian Shaman*. North Atlantic Books.

Luna, L. E., & White, S. F. (2000). *Ayahuasca Reader: Encounters with the Amazon's Sacred Vine*. Synergetic Press.

Mabit, J. (2007). Ayahuasca in the treatment of addictions. In M. J. Winkelman & T. B. Roberts (Eds.), *Psychedelic Medicine: New Evidence for Hallucinogenic Substances as Treatments* (Vol. 2, pp. 87–105). Praeger.

MacLean, K. A., Leoutsakos, J. M., Johnson, M. W., & Griffiths, R. R. (2012). Factor Analysis of the Mystical Experience Questionnaire: A Study of Experiences Occasioned by the Hallucinogen Psilocybin. *Journal for the Scientific Study of Religion, 51*(4), 721–737.

Malchiodi, C. A. (2003). *Handbook of Art Therapy*. The Guilford Press.

Malchiodi, C. A. (2015). *Creative Interventions with Traumatized Children*. Guilford Press.

Marlatt, G. A. (1996). Harm Reduction: Come as You Are. *Addictive Behaviors, 21*(6), 779–788.

Marwood, L., & Wise, T. (2017). Instability of Default Mode Network Connectivity in Major Depression: A Two-Sample Confirmation Study. *Translational Psychiatry*. Retrieved May 2, 2019, from https://www.nature.com/articles/tp201740

Mason, N. L., et al. (2020). Spontaneous and Deliberate Creative Cognition during and After Psilocybin Exposure. *Translational Psychiatry, 10*(1), 1–11.

May, G. G. (2004). *The Dark Night of the Soul: A Psychiatrist Explores the Connection Between Darkness and Spiritual Growth*. HarperCollins.

McCann, I. L., & Pearlman, L. A. (1990). Vicarious Traumatization: A Framework for Understanding the Psychological Effects of Working with Victims. *Journal of Traumatic Stress, 3*(1), 131–149.

McCraty, R., & Childre, D. (2010). Coherence: Bridging Personal, Social, and Global Health. *Alternative Therapies in Health and Medicine, 16*(4), 10–24.

McEvoy, M., & Ziegler, M. (2006). *Mindfulness-Based Cognitive Therapy for Depression*. Guilford Press.

McGilchrist, I. (2012). *The Master and His Emissary: The Divided Brain and the Making of the Western World*. Yale University Press.

McNiff, S. (1992). *Art as Medicine: Creating a Therapy of the Imagination*. Shambhala.

McNiff, S. (2004). *Art Heals: How Creativity Cures the Soul*. Shambhala.

Melnychuk, M. C., Dockree, P. M., O'Connell, R. G., Murphy, P. R., Balsters, J. H., & Robertson, I. H. (2018). Coupling of Respiration and Attention via the Locus Coeruleus: Effects of Meditation and Pranayama. *Psychophysiology, e13091*. https://doi.org/10.1111/psyp.13091

Metzner, R. (1999). *Sacred Vine of Spirits: Ayahuasca*. Park Street Press.

Metzner, R. (2004). *Sacred Mushroom of Visions: Teonanácatl*. Park Street Press.

Michaels, T. I., Purdon, J., Collins, A., et al. (2018). Inclusion of People of Color in Psychedelic-Assisted Psychotherapy: A Review of the Literature. *BMC Psychiatry, 18*(1), 245. https://doi.org/10.1186/s12888-018-1824-6

Miller, J. (2020). *The Psychedelic Renaissance: Legal and Ethical Considerations*. Psychedelic Science Press.

Mithoefer, M. C., et al. (2019). 3,4-Methylenedioxymethamphetamine (MDMA)-Assisted Therapy for Post-Traumatic Stress Disorder in Military Veterans, Firefighters, and Police Officers: A Randomized, Double-Blind, Dose-Response, Phase 2 Clinical Trial. *The Lancet Psychiatry, 5*(6), 486–497.

Mithoefer, M. C., Grob, C. S., & Brewerton, T. D. (2016). Novel Psychopharmacological Therapies for Psychiatric Disorders: Psilocybin and MDMA. *Lancet Psychiatry, 3*(5), 481–488.

Moody, R. A. (1975). *Life after Life*. Bantam.

Moon, B. L. (2002a). *Essentials of Art Therapy Education and Practice*. Charles C. Thomas Publisher.

Moon, B. L. (2002b). *The Dynamics of Art as Therapy with Adolescents*. Charles C Thomas Publisher, Ltd.

Moon, B. L. (2002c). *Working with Images: The Art of Art Therapists*. Charles C. Thomas Publisher.

Morgan, C. J. A., & Curran, H. V. (2011). Ketamine Use: A Review. *Addiction, 107*(1), 27–38.

Moss, R. (1996). *Conscious Dreaming: A Spiritual Path for Everyday Life*. Three Rivers Press.

Naumburg, M. (1987). *Dynamically Oriented Art Therapy: Its Principles and Practice*. Taylor & Francis.

Neff, K. D. (2003). Self-Compassion: An Alternative Conceptualization of a Healthy Attitude toward Oneself. *Self and Identity, 2*(2), 85–101.

Neff, K. D. (2011). *Self-Compassion: The Proven Power of Being Kind to Yourself*. HarperCollins.

Newberg, A., & Waldman, M. R. (2009). *How God Changes Your Brain: Breakthrough Findings from a Leading Neuroscientist*. Ballantine Books.

Nichols, D. E. (2016). Psychedelics. *Pharmacological Reviews, 68*(2), 264–355.

Nour, M. M., et al. (2016). Ego-Dissolution and Psychedelics: Validation of the Ego-Dissolution Inventory (EDI). *Frontiers in Human Neuroscience, 10*, 269. https://doi.org/10.3389/fnhum.2016.00269

Ogden, P. (2019). *Treating Trauma Master Series*. Retrieved on April 24, 2019, from https://www.nicabm.com/program/treating-trauma-master-4/?del=homepagepopular

Ogden, P., Minton, K., & Pain, C. (2006). *Trauma and the Body: A Sensorimotor Approach to Psychotherapy*. W.W. Norton & Company.

Parker, S. (2020). Trauma and Kundalini Yoga: A Critical Review of the Practice. *Journal of Yoga & Physical Therapy, 10*(1), 1–5.

Pennebaker, J. W. (1997). *Opening Up: The Healing Power of Expressing Emotions*. Guilford Press.

Perry, B. D., & Szalavitz, M. (2017). *The Boy Who Was Raised as a Dog: And Other Stories from a Child Psychiatrist's Notebook*. Basic Books.

Petri, G., et al. (2014). Homological Scaffolds of Brain Functional Networks. *Journal of the Royal Society Interface, 11*(101), 20140873.

Phelps, J. (2017). Developing Guidelines and Competencies for the Training of Psychedelic Therapists. *Journal of Humanistic Psychology, 57*(5), 450–487.

Pilecki, B., Luoma, J. B., Bathje, G. J., et al. (2021). Ethical and Legal Issues in Psychedelic Harm Reduction and Integration Therapy. *Harm Reduction Journal, 18*, 40. https://doi.org/10.1186/s12954-021-00489-1

Pollan, M. (2018). *How to Change Your Mind: What the New Science of Psychedelics Teaches Us about Consciousness, Dying, Addiction, Depression, and Transcendence.* Penguin Press.

Polster, E., & Polster, M. (1973). *Gestalt Therapy Integrated: Contours of Theory and Practice.* Brunner/Mazel.

Porges, S. W. (2011). *The Polyvagal Theory: Neurophysiological Foundations of Emotions, Attachment, Communication, and Self-Regulation.* W. W. Norton & Company.

Posner, J., Hellerstein, D. J., Gat, I., Mechling, A., Klahr, K., Wang, Z., McGrath, P. J., Stewart, J. W., & Peterson, B. S. (2013). Antidepressants Normalize the Default Mode Network in Patients with Dysthymia. *JAMA Psychiatry.* https://doi.org/10.1001/jamapsychiatry.2013.455

Proulx, L. (2017). *Attachment Informed Art Therapy: Strengthening Emotional Ties throughout the Lifetime.* Tellwell Talent

Raichle, M. E. (2015). The Brain's Default Mode Network. *Annual Review of Neuroscience, 38*, 433–447.

Raichle, M. E., et al. (2001). A Default Mode of Brain Function. *Proceedings of the National Academy of Sciences, 98*(2), 676–682.

Reich, D. L., Pichler, B., McKinney, R., & Duman, R. S. (2022). The "Psychedelic-Like" Effects of Ketamine. *Current Opinion in Psychiatry, 35*(1), 1–8.

Richards, W. A. (2015). *Sacred Knowledge: Psychedelics and Religious Experiences.* Columbia University Press.

Ring, K. (1982). *Life at Death: A Scientific Investigation of the Near-Death Experience.* William Morrow & Co.

Rosenberg, J. L., & Kitaen-Morse, B. (2004a). *The Body Speaks: The Role of Bodywork in Psychotherapy.* North Atlantic Books.

Rosenberg, J. L., & Kitaen-Morse, B. (2004b). *The Intimate Couple: Strengthening Love, Intimacy, and Commitment.* North Atlantic Books.

Rosenberg, J. L., Rand, M. L., & Asay, D. (1989). *Body, Self, and Soul: Sustaining Integration.* Humanics Limited.

Ross, S., et al. (2016). Rapid and Sustained Symptom Reduction Following Psilocybin Treatment for Anxiety and Depression in Patients with Life-Threatening Cancer: A Randomized Controlled Trial. *Journal of Psychopharmacology, 30*(12), 1165–1180.

Roth, G. (1998). *Maps to Ecstasy: A Healing Journey for the Untamed Spirit.* New World Library.

Roth, S., et al. (1997). *Childhood Trauma Remembered: A Report on the Current Scientific Knowledge Base and Its Applications.* American Psychological Association.

Rothschild, B. (2000). *The Body Remembers: The Psychophysiology of Trauma and Trauma Treatment.* W. W. Norton & Company.

Rubin, J. A. (2001). *Approaches to Art Therapy: Theory and Technique.* Brunner-Routledge.

Rubin, J. A. (2010). *Introduction to Art Therapy: Sources and Resources.* Routledge.

Ruck, C. A. P., Bigwood, J., Staples, D., Ott, J., & Wasson, R. G. (1979). Entheogens. *Journal of Psychedelic Drugs, 11*(1–2), 145–146.

Sannella, L. (1987). *Kundalini: Psychosis or Transcendence?* Integral Publishing.

Saraswati, S. (1984). *Asana, Pranayama, Mudra, Bandha.* Bihar School of Yoga.

Saunders, N., & Doblin, R. (1996). Psychedelic research in the United Kingdom. *MAPS Bulletin, 6*(1), 32–35.

Schaverien, J. (1992). *The Revealing Image: Analytical Art Psychotherapy in Theory and Practice*. Tavistock/Routledge.

Schore, A. N. (2003). *Affect Dysregulation and Disorders of the Self*. W.W. Norton & Company.

Schore, A. N. (2012). *The Science of the Art of Psychotherapy*. Norton.

Schore, A. N. (2019). *The Development of the Unconscious Mind*. W. W. Norton & Company.

Schultes, R. E., & Hofmann, A. (1980). *The Botany and Chemistry of Hallucinogens*. Charles C. Thomas Publisher.

Schwartz, R. (2020a). *Internal Family Systems Therapy* (2nd ed.). Guilford Press.

Schwartz, R. (2020b). *No Bad Parts: Healing Trauma and Restoring Wholeness with the Internal Family Systems Model*. Sounds True.

Schwartz, R., & Falconer, R. (2021). *Many Minds, One Self: Evidence for a Radical Shift in Paradigm*. Chiron Publications.

Scott, D. (2015). *The Complete Guide to Internal Family Systems Therapy*. CreateSpace Independent Publishing Platform.

Scott, D. (2021). *Addiction and the Internal Family Systems Model*. SAGE Publishing.

Scott, D. (2022a). *Internal Family Systems Therapy for Healing Trauma*. Self-published.

Scott, D. (2022b). *The Therapist's Guide to IFS: How to Integrate Internal Family Systems into Your Practice*. PESI Publishing.

Scott-Alexander, M. (2023). *The Just Right Next: A Book of Emergent Poems*. iUniverse.

Sessa, B. (2012). Shaping the Renaissance of Psychedelic Research. *The Lancet, 380*(9838), 200–201. https://doi.org/10.1016/S0140-6736(12)60600-X

Sessa, B. (2017). *The Psychedelic Renaissance: Reassessing the Role of Psychedelic Drugs in 21st Century Psychiatry and Society*. Muswell Hill Press.

Shanon, B. (2002). *The Antipodes of the Mind: Charting the Phenomenology of the Ayahuasca Experience*. Oxford University Press.

Shanon, B. (2010). The Epistemics of Ayahuasca Visions. *Phenomenology and the Cognitive Sciences, 9*(2), 263–280. https://doi.org/10.1007/s11097-010-9161-3

Shaver, P. R., & Mikulincer, M. (2012). *Attachment in Adulthood: Structure, Dynamics, and Change*. Guilford Press.

Sheline, Y. I., Barch, D. M., Price, J. L., Rundle, M. M., Vaishnavi, S. N., Snyder, A. Z., Mintun, M. A., Wang, S., Coalson, R. S., & Raichle, M. E. (2019). The Default Mode Network and Self-Referential Processes in Depression. *PNAS, 106*(6), 1942–1947. https://doi.org/10.1073/pnas.0812686106

Shulgin, A., & Shulgin, A. (1991). *PIHKAL: A Chemical Love Story*. Transform Press.

Siegel, D. J. (2010a). *Mindsight: The New Science of Personal Transformation*. Bantam.

Siegel, D. J. (2010b). *The Mindful Therapist: A Clinician's Guide to Mindsight and Neural Integration*. W.W. Norton & Company.

Siegel, D. J. (2012). *The Developing Mind: How Relationships and the Brain Interact to Shape Who We Are*. Guilford Press.

Siegel, D. J., & Hartzell, M. (2014). *Parenting from the Inside Out: How a Deeper Self-Understanding Can Help You Raise Children Who Thrive*. TarcherPerigee.

Simpson, A. (2017). *The Other Side of Eden: Hunters, Farmers, and the Shaping of the World*. North Atlantic Books.

Smith, H. (2000). *Cleansing the Doors of Perception: The Religious Significance of Entheogenic Plants and Chemicals*. Tarcher/Putnam.

Smith, H. (2017). *Peyote and Other Psychoactive Cacti*. Ronin Publishing.

Smith, L. T. (2012). *Decolonizing Methodologies: Research and Indigenous Peoples*. Zed Books.

Stark, R., & Bainbridge, W. S. (1985). *The Future of Religion: Secularization, Revival, and Cult Formation.* University of California Press.

Stewart, O. C. (1987). *Peyote Religion: A History.* University of Oklahoma Press.

Strassman, R. (2001). *DMT: The Spirit Molecule.* Park Street Press.

Swami Sivananda Radha. (1990). *Realities of the Dreaming Mind: The Practice of Dream Yoga.* Timeless Books.

Tafur, J. (2017). *Fellowship of the River: A Medical Doctor's Exploration into Traditional Amazonian Plant Medicine.* Espiritu Books.

Tart, C. T. (1972). *States of Consciousness.* E. P. Dutton.

Tart, C. T. (1990). *Psi: Scientific Studies of the Psychic Realm.* Pargament Books.

Tedlock, B. (2005). *The Woman in the Shaman's Body: Reclaiming the Feminine in Religion and Medicine.* Bantam.

Terence McKenna. (1992). *Food of the Gods: The Search for the Original Tree of Knowledge.* Bantam Books.

Thompson, E. (2020). *Waking, Dreaming, Being: Self and Consciousness in Neuroscience, Meditation, and Philosophy.* Columbia University Press.

Trinity College Dublin. (2018a, May 10). The Yogi Masters Were Right—Meditation and Breathing Exercises Can Sharpen Your Mind: New Research Explains Link Between Breath-Focused Meditation and Attention and Brain Health. *ScienceDaily.* Retrieved April 28, 2019, from https://www.sciencedaily.com/releases/2018/05/180510101254.htm

Trinity College Dublin. (2018b). *The Neuroscience of Mindfulness Meditation.* Trinity College Dublin Press.

Tupper, K. W. (2002). Entheogens and Existential Intelligence: The Use of Plant Teachers as Cognitive Tools. *Canadian Journal of Education, 27*(4), 499–516.

Tupper, K. W. (2008). The Globalization of Ayahuasca: Harm Reduction or Benefit Maximization? *International Journal of Drug Policy, 19*(4), 297–303.

Tupper, K. W. (2009). Entheogenic Healing: The Spiritual Effects and Therapeutic Potential of Ceremonial Ayahuasca Use. *The Canadian Journal of Native Studies, 29*(1/2), 57–83.

Turner, V. (1969). *The Ritual Process: Structure and Anti-Structure.* Aldine Publishing.

Tylš, F., Páleníček, T., & Horáček, J. (2014). Psilocybin – Summary of Knowledge and New Perspectives. *European Neuropsychopharmacology, 24*(3), 342–356.

Underhill, E. (1911). *Mysticism: A Study in the Nature and Development of Spiritual Consciousness.* E. P. Dutton.

van der Kolk, B. A. (2014). *The Body Keeps the Score: Brain, Mind, and Body in the Healing of Trauma.* Viking.

Volpi-Abadie, J., Kaye, A. M., & Kaye, A. D. (2013). Serotonin Syndrome. *Ochsner Journal, 13*(4), 533–540.

Wallace, A. F. C. (2003). *Religion: An Anthropological View.* Random House.

Wallace, K. (2024, January 8–February 26). *Internal Family Systems (IFS) Practice & Process Workshop* [Workshop]. Caravan Counselling.

Walsh, R. (2007). *The World of Shamanism: New Views of an Ancient Tradition.* Llewellyn Publications.

Walsh, R. N., & Shapiro, S. L. (2006). The Meeting of Meditative Disciplines and Western Psychology: A Mutually Enriching Dialogue. *American Psychologist, 61*(3), 227–239. https://doi.org/10.1037/0003-066X.61.3.227

Wasson, R. G. (1980). *The Wondrous Mushroom: Mycolatry in Mesoamerica.* McGraw-Hill.

Watts, A. (1966). *The Book: On the Taboo Against Knowing Who You Are.* Vintage Books.

Watts, R., Day, C., Krzanowski, J., Nutt, D., & Carhart-Harris, R. (2017). Patients' Accounts of Increased "Connectedness" and "Acceptance" After Psilocybin for Treatment-Resistant Depression. *Journal of Humanistic Psychology, 57*(5), 520–564.

Wilber, K. (2001). *A Brief History of Everything*. Shambhala.

Wilcox, J. A., Evans, W. E., & Freeman, T. L. (2014). The Potential for Serotonin Syndrome Following Psychedelic Ingestion. *Journal of Psychoactive Drugs, 46*(2), 126–133.

Wilson, S. (2008). *Research Is Ceremony: Indigenous Research Methods*. Fernwood Publishing.

Winkelman, M. (2010). *Shamanism: A Biopsychosocial Paradigm of Consciousness and Healing*. Praeger.

Woolfe, S. (n.d.). *When does psychedelic use become a form of escapism?* Webdelics. Retrieved January 31, 2025, from https://www.webdelics.com/post/psychedelic-use-escapism

Woolley, J. D. (2017). Psychedelic-Assisted Therapy: A Review of the Literature. *Journal of Psychoactive Drugs, 49*(1), 26–37.

Zarate, C. A., Singh, J. B., Carlson, P. J., Brutsche, N. E., Ameli, R., Luckenbaugh, D. A., Charney, D. S., & Manji, H. K. (2006). A Randomized Trial of an N-Methyl-D-Aspartate Antagonist in Treatment-Resistant Major Depression. *Archives of General Psychiatry, 63*(8), 856–864. https://doi.org/10.1001/archpsyc.63.8.856

Zendo Project. (n.d.). *Psychedelic Peer Support*. Retrieved from Zendo Project website: https://zendoproject.org

Zinberg, N. E. (1984). *Drug, Set, and Setting: The Basis for Controlled Intoxicant Use*. Yale University Press.

Znamenski, A. (2007). *The Beauty of the Primitive: Shamanism and the Western Imagination*. Oxford University Press.

Suggested Reading

The following works have influenced the content of this book but were not directly cited in the text. They are included here as suggested reading for those interested in further exploring this topic.

Aixala, M. (2022). *Psychedelic Integration: Psychotherapy for Non-Ordinary States of Consciousness*. Synergetic Press.

Alarcon, D. (2023). Cave paintings and psychedelics. *Art 525/Art History 5290 Papers, 18*. https://scholarworks.lib.csusb.edu/art-history-papers/18

AlFardan, S., Rose, J., Siddig, M., & Yousif, A. (n.d.). Psychedelics for Post-Traumatic Stress Disorder: A Systematic Review and Meta-Analysis. *Journal of Nervous and Mental Disease*. h

Allen, J. (n.d.). Psychedelic Integration Art Therapist. *Bone Knowing*. Retrieved August 16, 2024, from https://boneknowing.com/

American Psychiatric Association. (2013). *Diagnostic and Statistical Manual of Mental Disorders* (5th ed.). American Psychiatric Publishing.

Berlant, S. R. (2005). The Entheomycological Origin of Egyptian Crowns and the Esoteric Underpinnings of Egyptian Religion. *Journal of Ethnopharmacology, 102*(2), 275–288. https://doi.org/10.1016/j.jep.2005.07.028

California Institute of Integral Studies. (n.d.). *Certificate in Psychedelic Therapy and Research*. Retrieved August 16, 2024, from https://www.ciis.edu/research-centers-and-initiatives/center-for-psychedelic-therapies-and-research

Center for Mindfulness Medicine. (n.d.). *Allison and Daniel McQueen*. Retrieved August 16, 2024, from https://medicinalmindfulness.org/therapists-and-guides/

Colcott, J., Guerin, A. A., Carter, O. et al. (2024). Side-Effects of MDMA-Assisted Psychotherapy: A Systematic Review and Meta-Analysis. *Neuropsychopharmacology, 49*, 1208–1226. https://doi.org/10.1038/s41386-024-01865-8

Curtis, R., Roberts, L., Graves, E., Rainey, H. T., Wynn, D., Krantz, D., & Wieloch, V. (2020). The Role of Psychedelics and Counseling in Mental Health Treatment. *Journal of Mental Health Counseling, 42*(4), 323–338.

Denning, P., & Little, J. (2024). *Practicing Harm Reduction Psychotherapy.* Guilford Publications.

Dreamflesh. (n.d.). *Rock Art & Psychedelics.* Retrieved August 16, 2024, from https://dreamflesh.com/essay/rock-art-psychedelic/

Enders, C. (2024). How Psychedelic Drug Research Got High on Its Own Supply. *New York Times.* Retrieved August 25, 2024. https://www.nytimes.com/2024/08/23/opinion/psychedelics-mdma-mental-health.html

Erowid. (n.d.). *Documenting the Complex Relationship between Humans and Psychoactives.* Retrieved August 16, 2024, from https://www.erowid.org/

Fisher, J., & Ogden, P. (2015). *Sensorimotor Psychotherapy: Interventions for Trauma and Attachment.* W.W. Norton & Company.

Glue, P., Loo, C., Fam, J. et al. (2024). Extended-release Ketamine Tablets for Treatment-resistant Depression: A Randomized Placebo-controlled Phase 2 Trial. *Nature Medicine, 30,* 2004–2009. https://doi.org/10.1038/s41591-024-03063-x

Grof, S. (2019). *The Way of the Psychonaut Volume One and Two: Encyclopedia for Inner Journeys.* Multidisciplinary Association for Psychedelic Studies.

Grof, S., & Grof, C. (1989). *Spiritual Emergency: When Personal Transformation Becomes a Crisis.* Tarcher Perigee.

Guerra-Doce, E. (2015). Psychoactive Substances in Prehistoric Times: Examining the Archaeological Evidence. *Time and Mind, 8*(1), 91–112.

Husum, C. (2022). *Psychedelic Integration for A Life Transformed* (2nd ed.). Retrieved August 16, 2024, from https://courses.centreoftheheart.com/p/psychedelic-integration-full-course-modules-1-8

Janiger, O., & De Rios, M. D. (1989). LSD and Creativity. *Journal of Psychoactive Drugs, 21*(1), 129–134.

Johnson, R. A. (1991). *Owning Your Own Shadow: Understanding the Dark Side of the Psyche.* HarperSanFrancisco.

Kedar, Y., Kedar, G., & Barkai, R. (2021). Hypoxia in Paleolithic Decorated Caves: The Use of Artificial Light in Deep Caves Reduces Oxygen Concentration and induces Altered States of Consciousness. *Time and Mind, 14*(2), 181–216. https://doi.org/10.1080/1751696X.2021.1903177

Ketamine Training Center. (n.d.). *Training in Ketamine-Assisted Therapy.* Retrieved August 16, 2024, from https://theketaminetrainingcenter.com/

Khalsa, S. B. (2006). Meditation as a Therapeutic Intervention: A Brief Review. *Clinical Neurophysiology, 22*(2), 73–78.

Leone, L. et al. (2024). Psychedelics and Evidence-based Psychotherapy: A Systematic Review with Recommendations for Advancing Psychedelic Therapy Research. *Psychiatric Clinics of North America, 47*(2), 367–398. https://doi.org/10.1016/J.PSC.2024.02.006

Lii, T. R., Smith, A. E., Flohr, J. R. et al. (2023). Randomized Trial of Ketamine Masked by Surgical Anesthesia in Patients with Depression. *Nature Mental Health, 1,* 876–886. https://doi.org/10.1038/s44220-023-00140-x

Lowy, B. (1971). New Records of Mushroom Stones from Guatemala. *Mycologia, 63*(5), 983–993.

Microdose Buzz. (2021, July 1). Ancient Civilizations and Psychedelics. *Microdose.* Retrieved August 16, 2024, from https://microdose.buzz/news/ancient-civilizations-and-psychedelics/

National Geographic. (2021, July 27). 400 Years Ago, Visitors Painted a Cave—and Took Hallucinogens. *National Geographic*. Retrieved August 16, 2024, from https://www.nationalgeographic.com/science/article/400-years-ago-visitors-painted-cave-took-hallucinogens

Nhất, H., Ho, M., & Vo-Dinh, M. (1987). *The Miracle of Mindfulness: An Introduction to the Practice of Meditation*. Beacon Press.

Nutt, D., Erritzoe, D., & Carhart-Harris, R. (2020). Psychedelic psychiatry's brave new world. *Cell, 181*(1), 24–28. https://doi.org/10.1016/j.cell.2020.02.016

Perkins, A. M., Arnone, D., Smallwood, J., & Mobbs, D. (2015). Thinking Too Much: Self-Generated thought as the Engine of Neuroticism. *Trends in Cognitive Sciences, 19*(9), 492–498.

Pinchbeck, D. (2002). *Breaking Open the Head: A Psychedelic Journey into the Heart of Contemporary Shamanism*. Broadway Books.

Psychedelic Spotlight. (2021, July 1). 5 Examples of Ancient Psychedelic Cave Art. *Psychedelic Spotlight*. Retrieved August 16, 2024, from https://psychedelicspotlight.com/5-examples-of-ancient-psychedelic-cave-art/

Psychedelic Support. (n.d.). A List of Therapists Who Help Clients Integrate Psychedelic Experiences. *Psychedelic Support*. Retrieved August 16, 2024, from https://psychedelic.support/

Read, T., & Papaspyrou, M. (Eds.). (2021). *Psychedelics and Psychotherapy: The Healing Potential of Expanded States*. Simon and Schuster.

Riley, D., & O'Hare, P. (2000). Harm Reduction: History, Definition, and Practice. In L. D. Harrison & J. A. Inciardi (Eds.), *Harm Reduction: National and International Perspectives* (1st edn). Sage Publications. pp. 1–26.

Rosenberg, J. L., & Morse, B. K. (1987). *Integrative Body Psychotherapy: Towards a New Understanding of the Whole Person*. North Atlantic Books.

Savary, L. M., Berne, P. H., & Kaplan-Williams, S. (1984). *Dreams and Spiritual Growth: A Christian Approach to Dreamwork*. Paulist Press.

Schenberg, E. E. (2018). Psychedelic-Assisted Psychotherapy: A Paradigm Shift in Psychiatric Research and Development. *Frontiers in Pharmacology, 9*, 733.

Schultes, R. E. (1969). Hallucinogens of Plant Origin: Interdisciplinary Studies of Plants Sacred in Primitive Cultures Yield Results of Academic and Practical Interest. *Science, 163*(3864), 245–254.

Sevelius, J. (2019). How Psychedelic Science Privileges Some, Neglects Others, and Limits Us All [Internet]. *Chacruna*. Retrieved October 30, 2020, from https://chacruna.net/how-psychedelic-science-privileges-some-neglects-others/

Stein, M. (1998). *Jung's Map of the Soul: An Introduction*. Open Court.

Teixeira, P. J., Johnson, M. W., Timmermann, C., Watts, R., Erritzoe, D., Douglass, H., Kettner, H., & Carhart-Harris, R. L. (2022). Psychedelics and Health Behaviour Change. *Journal of Psychopharmacology, 36*(1), 12–19. https://doi.org/10.1177/02698811211008554

University of Nevada, Reno. (2021, May 14). Indigenous Americans took hallucinogens 400 years ago. *Nevada Today*. Retrieved August 16, 2024, from https://www.unr.edu/nevada-today/news/2021/indigenous-americans-took-hallucinogens

UPI. (2011, March 7). Cave Art May Show Magic Mushrooms. *UPI*. https://www.upi.com/Science_News/2011/03/07/Cave-art-may-show-magic-mushrooms/UPI-70561299548511/

Wikipedia. (n.d.). *Lascaux Painting*. Retrieved August 16, 2024, from https://upload.wikimedia.org/wikipedia/commons/1/1e/Lascaux_painting.jpg

INDEX

Note: *Italic* page numbers refer to figures.